Ultrasound Teaching Manual

The Basics of Performing and Interpreting Ultrasound Scans

Matthias Hofer, M.D.

With the collaboration of
Tatjana Reihs, M.D.

Translated by
Peter F. Winter, M.D.

486 Illustrations

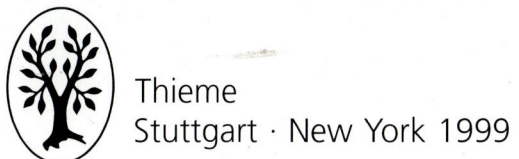

Thieme
Stuttgart · New York 1999

Matthias Hofer, M.D.
Institute for Diagnostic Radiology
(Chairman: Prof. U. Mödder, M.D.)
H. Heine University
Düsseldorf, Germany

Tatjana Reihs, M.D.
Department of Obstetrics and Gynecology
H. Heine University
Düsseldorf, Germany

Translated by
Peter F. Winter, M.D.
Chlinical Professor of Radiology
Boston University
School of Medicine,
Clinical Assistant Professor
University of Illinois
College of Medicine at Peoria
USA

Library of Congress Cataloging-in-Publication Data

Hofer, Matthias.
 [Sono Grundkurs.   English]
  Ultrasound Teaching Manual, The Basics of Performing and Interpreting Ultrasound Scans / Matthias Hofer : translated by Peter F. Winter.
  p.   cm.
  Rev. translation of: Sono Grundkurs. 1997.
  Includes bibliographical references and index.
  ISBN 3-13-111041-4. — ISBN 0-86577-725-X (TNY)
  1. Diagnosis. Ultrasonic.   I. Title.
  [DNLM: 1. Ultrasonography,   WN 208 H697s 1999]
RC78.7.U4H6413   1999
616.07'543—dc21
DNLM/DLC
for Library of Congress   98-45748
                                                             CIP

Some of the product names, patents, and registered designs referred to in this book are in fact registered trademarks or proprietary names even though specific reference to this fact is not always made in the text. Therefore, the appearance of a name without designation as proprietary is not to be construed as a representation by the publisher that it is in the public domain.

This book, including all parts thereof, is legally protected by copyright. Any use, exploitation or commercialization outside the narrow limits set by copyright legislation, without the publisher's consent, is illegal and liable to prosecution. This applies in particular to photostat reproduction, copying, mimeographing or duplication of any kind, translating, preparation of microfilms, and electronic data processing and storage.

© 1999 Georg Thieme Verlag, Rüdigerstraße 14,
D-70469 Stuttgart, Germany
Thieme New York, 333 Seventh Avenue,
New York, NY 10001, USA

Typesetting by primustype R. Hurler GmbH,
D-73274 Notzingen
typeset on Textline/HerculesPro
Printed in Germany by Druckhaus Götz, Ludwigsburg

ISBN 3-13-111041-4 (GTV)
ISBN 0-86577-725-X (TNY)   1 2 3 4 5 6

List of Abbreviations

AC	Abdominal circumference
ASD	Atrial septal defect
BPD	Biparietal diameter
CRL	Crown-rump length
CT	Computed tomography
d_{AO}	Diameter of the aorta
d_{VC}	Diameter of the inferior vena cava
EFW	Estimated fetal weight
EP	Ectopic pregnancy
ERCP	Endoscopic retrograde cholangiopancreatography
ESWL	Extracorporeal shock wave lithotripsy
FHVI	Frontal horn ventricular index
FL	Femoral length
FNH	Focal nodular hyperplasia
GI	Gastrointestinal tract
GSD	Gestational sac (= chorionic cavity) diameter
HC	Head circumference
HCG	Human chorionic gonadotropin
IUD	Intrauterine device
IVF	In vitro fertilization
MCL	Midclavicular line
MRI	Magnetic resonance imaging
NPO	Nothing by mouth
NT	Nuchal translucency
OFD	Occipitofrontal diameter
OHVI	Occipital horn ventricular index
PCOS	Polycystic ovarian syndrome
PW	Pulsed wave Doppler
RI	Resistance index
SLE	Systemic lupus erythematosus
SMA	Superior mesenteric artery
S/P	Status post
TGA	Transposition of the great arteries
Vol_{ub}	Volume of the urinary bladder
VSD	Ventricular septal defect
YSD	Yolk sac diameter

Important Note:

Medicine is an ever-changing science undergoing continual development. Research and clinical experience are continually expanding our knowledge, in particular our knowledge of proper treatment and drug therapy. Insofar as this book mentions any dosage or application, readers may rest assured that the authors, editors, and publishers have made every effort to ensure that such references are in accordance with **the state of knowledge at the time of production of the book.**

Nevertheless, this does not involve, imply, or express any guarantee or responsibility on the part of the publishers in respect of any dosage instructions and forms of application stated in the book. **Every user is requested to examine carefully** the manufacturer's leaflets accompanying each drug and to check, if necessary in consultation with a physician or specialist, whether the dosage schedules mentioned therein or the contraindications stated by the manufacturers differ from the statements made in the present book. Such examination is particularly important with drugs that are either rarely used or have been newly released on the market. **Every dosage schedule or every form of application used is entirely at the user's own risk and responsibility.** The authors and publishers request every user to report to the publishers any discrepancies or inaccuracies noticed.

Foreword

The increasing role that imaging procedures have assumed in the clinical routine must be considered at an early stage in the education of medical students. The vast use and non-invasive character of sonography make it prudent to familiarize tomorrow's physicians today with this comparatively low-risk technology.

The pilot project on medical didactics that began in Düsseldorf in 1992 consisted of preliminary lessons in sonography for a few medical students particularly interested in sonography and endoscopy. Soon, the hands-on instructions in small groups became more and more accepted and this teaching concept could be enlarged and improved.

Under the guidance of residents and lecturers, student instructors relate the sonographic diagnostic to their junior students. The participants examine each other and systematically learn the anatomic relationship of the abdominal organs as seen in the standard sonographic sections. Step by step, they learn how to use and handle the transducer. These hands-on instructions are accompanied by complementary lectures, which address the subject of differential diagnosis of the pathologic changes by means of videos, slides, and live demonstrations.

The workbook presented here is largely based on the curriculum of this introductory sonography course for beginners. The approach selected here considers in particular the difficulties generally encountered by the novice. By relying on the step-by-step process of the workbook, the novice will soon realize that initial frustration ("I only see a snow storm") will soon give way to increasing enthusiasm for this elegant modality.

It should be pointed out, however, that each sonographic diagnosis can only be as good as the examiner. False diagnoses can only be avoided through profound anatomic and sonomorphologic knowledge, unrelenting thoroughness, and, where appropriate, comparison with other imaging procedures. Intitial successes ("I now recognize all parenchymal organs") should not lead to overconfidence during the learning phase; a truly profound knowledge can only be gained through long exposure in the clinical setting and the resultant practical experience that leads to the familiarization of the diverse anatomic variations and pathologic changes.

This workbook, of course, cannot encompass all aspects of diagnostic sonography and this is not its goal. Instead, it should offer the reader an optimal introduction to sonography. The spectrum of the information presented and the pathologic examples are especially targeted at the beginner. The carefully prepared didactic presentation, which reflects the author's teaching experience over many years, will hopefully motivate or perhaps even excite many students.

Düsseldorf

Ulrich Mödder, M.D.
Director, Institute of Diagnostic Radiology
Heinrich-Heine-University, Düsseldorf
Germany

Introduction and Suggestions to the Reader

This workbook is primarily for medical students, technicians, and residents that have had no or little exposure to sonography and wish to learn this technique systematically. The first step is recognizing the normal anatomic structures.

Each section therefore begins with the anatomic orientation of the respective body region (where is the top of the image?) before presenting and commenting on a selection of the most common diseases.

Before reading the individual sections, the material on pages 6 to 10 should be studied to learn the basics **before** the hands-on practice. Thereafter, it is advisable to make a drawing of the body planes as seen in typical longitudinal (sagittal) as well as in typical cross (transverse) sections, for example on a cone coffee filter. The shape of the cone coffee filter corresponds to the shape of the sonographic image for the examination of the abdomen.

At this stage the reader can already experience the gratification of successful learning. The correct answer should **not be passively** copied from page 78. Instead, the anterior and dorsal structures as well as the superior and inferior structures, as seen on the sagittal section and viewed from the patient's right side, **should be deduced**. The cone coffee filter should be placed on the abdomen and oriented along the plane of the sonographic beam of a transducer (convex border of the cone coffee filter) placed on the epigastric region along the midline (linea alba, between both rectus muscles) **(Fig. 4.1 a)**.

Next, anterior and dorsal structures as well as right and left structures should be marked on the reverse of the cone coffee filter as seen on the cross-sectional (transverse) sonographic image viewed from below (!) **(Fig. 4.1 b)**. Only after mastering the spatial orientation is the reader prepared for studying the normal findings as seen in the standard planes and, thereafter, the diffuse and focal abnormalities of the individual organs.

An explanatory diagram, intentionally annotated with numbers only, is placed adjacent to each sonographic image, facilitating the interpretation of the sonographic image with the help of numbers incorporated in the accompanying text. To confirm the interpretation after the text has been studied, the back cover can be opened to use the key found on the unfolded cover page. By blocking the labels, it is easy to check whether all structures have been correctly identified. The numbers of the labels apply to all the diagrams in this workbook.

If the thirst for knowledge has not yet been quenched, the quiz found at the end of each section can be tackled. The images in the quiz should be identified as to sectional orientation and visualized structures, and, if possible, a differential diagnosis provided. Only afterwards should the answers on pages 76 and 77 be consulted since the suspense is prematurely lost otherwise. The quiz may possibly arouse diagnostic inquisitiveness and lead to a first feeling of achievement through an imaging procedure. Whenever these practical applications do not readily lend a mental concept of the imaging plane in question or the reader is confronted with other discouraging events, help may be found on pages 78 and 79.

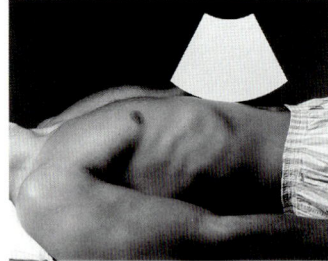 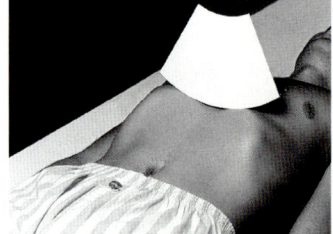

Fig. 4.1 a   **Fig. 4.1 b**

Contents

Image Formation and Echogenicity
Operating Sonographic Equipment 7
**Sonographic Equipment and Selection of the
Appropriate Transducer** 8
Artifacts 9

1 Sagittal Overview

Upper Retroperitoneum 11
Lower Retroperitoneum in Oblique Sections: Normal
Findings 12
Aortic Ectasia and Aneurysms 13
Retroperitoneum: Lymph Nodes 14
Retroperitoneum: Other Clinical Cases 15

2 Axial Overview

Upper Abdomen: Basic Anatomy 17
Upper Abdomen: Normal Findings 18
Upper Abdomen: Pancreatitis 19
Pancreas: Additional Cases 20
Upper Abdomen: Lymph Nodes 21
Quiz for Self-Assessment 22

3 Liver

Porta Hepatis: Normal Findings 23
Portal Hypertension: Lymph Nodes 24
Hepatic Vein Confluence and Hepatic Congestion 25
Hepatic Size, Gallbladder, Normal Findings 26
Normal Variants, Fatty Liver 27
Focal Fatty Infiltration 28
Other Focal Changes 29
Infections, Parasite 30
Cirrhosis and Hepatocellular Carcinoma 31
Hepatic Metastases 32
Quiz for Self-Assessment 33

4 Gallbladder and Biliary Ducts

Cholestasis 34
Gallstones and Polyps 35
Cholecystitis and Quiz for Self-Assessment 36

5 Kidneys and Adrenal Glands

Normal Findings 37
Normal Variants and Cysts 38
Atrophy and Inflammation 39
Urinary Obstruction 40
Differential Diagnosis of Urinary Obstruction 41
Renal Stones and Infarcts 42
Renal Tumors 43
Renal Transplant: Normal Findings 44
Renal Transplant 45
Quiz for Self-Assessment 46

6 Spleen

Normal Findings 47
Diffuse Splenomegaly 48
Focal Splenic Changes 49
Quiz for Self-Assessment 50

7 GI Tract

Stomach 51
Colon 52
Small Bowel 53

8 Urinary Bladder

Normal Findings, Volume Measurements 54
Indwelling Catheter, Cystitis, Sediment 55

9 Male Genital Organs

Prostate Gland, Testicles and Scrotum 56
Undescended Testicle, Orchitis/Epididymitis 57

10 Female Genital Organs

Normal Findings 58
Uterus 59
Tumors of the Uterus 60
Ovaries 61

11 Pregnancy

Diagnosis of Early Pregnancy 63
Biometry In the First Trimester 64
Biometry In the Second and Third Trimester 65
Placental Location and Fetal Gender 66
Diagnosis of Fetal Malformations 67
Quiz for Self-Assessment 73

12 Thyroid Gland

Normal Findings 74
Diffuse and Focal Changes 75

Solutions to the Quiz 76
Tips and Tricks for the Beginner 78
Acknowledgement 80

On the fold-out covers:
Front: **Standard Sonographic Sections**
Rear: **Index**
Key to Diagrams
Normal Measurements

Image Formation and Echogenicity

The sonographic image begins with mechanical oscillations of a crystal that has been excited by electrical pulses (piezoelectric effect). These oscillations are emitted as sound waves from the crystals **(dark blue arrows)** just as sound waves are emitted from a loudspeaker membrane **(Fig. 6.1)**, though the frequencies used in sonography are not audible to the human ear. Depending on the desired application, the sonographic frequencies range from 2.0 to approximately 15.0 MHz. Several crystals are assembled to form a transducer from which sound waves propagate through the tissues, to be reflected and returned as echoes **(light blue arrows)** to the transducer. The returning echoes are, in reverse, converted by the crystals into electrical pulses that are then used to compute the sonographic image.

The sound waves are reflected at the interfaces **(A, B, C)** between media of different acoustic density (i.e., different sound propagation). The reflection of the sound waves is proportionate to the difference in acoustic density: a moderate difference **(interface A in Fig. 6.1a)** will reflect and return a portion of the sound beam to the transducer, with the remaining sound waves to be transmitted and propagated further into deeper tissue layers.

If the difference in acoustic density increases **(interface B in Fig. 6.1b)**, the intensity of the reflected sound also increases, and that of the transmitted sound decreases proportionately. If the acoustic densities are vastly different **(interface B in Fig. 6.1b)**, the sound beam is completely reflected and total acoustic shadowing **(45)** results (total reflection). Acoustic shadowing is observed behind bone (ribs), stones (in kidneys or the gallbladder), and air (intestinal gas).

Figure 6.3 illustrates acoustic shadowing **(45)** behind an air-containing bowel loop **(46)**. Echoes are not elicited if no differences in acoustic density are encountered: homogeneous fluids (blood, bile, urine, and cyst content, but also ascites and pleural effusion) are seen as echo-free (black) structures, e.g., the gallbladder **(14)** and hepatic vessels **(10, 11)** in **Figure 6.3**.

The processor computes the depth from which the echo originated from the registered temporal difference between emission of the sound beam pulse and reception of the echo. Echoes from tissues close to the transducer **(A)** arrive earlier (t_A) than echoes from deeper tissues (t_B, t_C) **(Fig. 6.1)**.

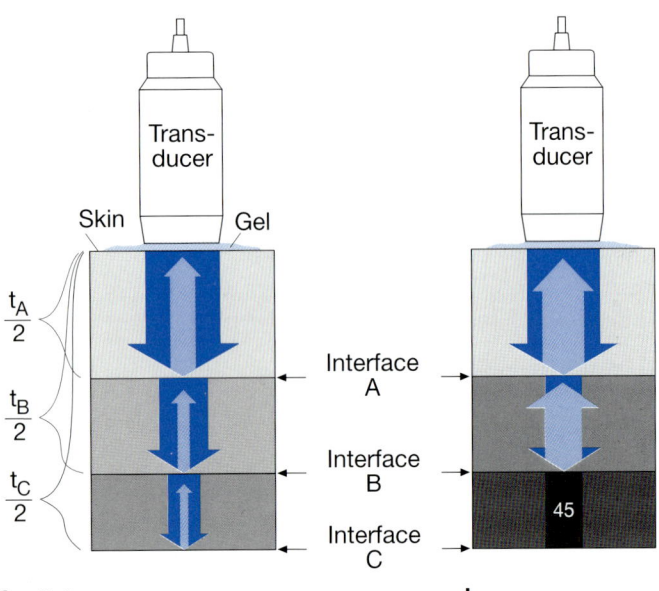

Fig. 6.1 a   **b**

An echo reflected repeatedly back and forth **(Fig. 6.2)** before it returns to the transducer has a travel time that is no longer proportionate to the distance of its origin. The processor incorrectly assigns these reverberation echoes **(51)** to a deeper level **(Fig. 10.1)**.

Additional distortion occurs through propagation speed errors introduced by programming the processor based on the assumption that the propagation speed of sound in tissue is constant, whereas in actual fact it is different for each type of tissue. While sound travels through the liver with a speed of about 1570 m/sec, it travels through fat with a lower speed of 1476 m/sec. The assumed medium speed stored in the processor leads to small differences but no major distortion.

If the propagation speed of adjacent tissue is vastly different (bone: 3360 m/sec vs. air: 331 m/sec), total reflection takes place **(Fig. 6.1b along interface B)** and acoustic shadowing ensues **(45)**. For this reason a coupling gel is needed to assure direct contact between transducer and skin, with no air trapped in between.

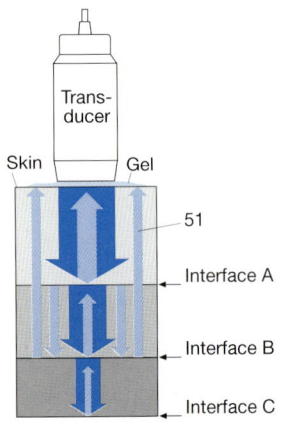

Fig. 6.2

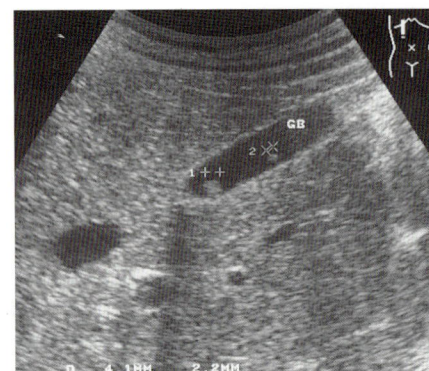

Fig. 6.3 a

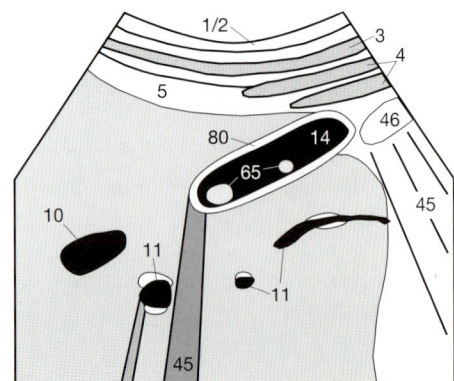

Fig. 6.3 b

Operating Sonographic Equipment

The steps relevant for operating a sonographic unit are introduced here by means of a medium-sized unit (Toshiba). First, the patient's name has to be entered correctly **(A, B)** for proper identification. The keys for changing the program **(C)** or transducer **(D)** are found on the upper half of the control panel.

On most panels the freeze button **(E)** is in the right lower corner. When activated, this will prevent the real-time images from changing. We recommend having one finger of the left hand always resting on this button, thus minimizing any delay in freezing the desired image for measuring, annotating, or printing. The overall amplification of the received echoes is controlled by the gain knob **(F)**.

Depth gain compensation: For selective enhancement of echoes received from different depths, the amplication can also be selectively adjusted with slide-pots **(G)** to compensate for depth-related losses in signal. Moving the image depth up or down, usually in small increments, increases or deceases the field of view **(I)**. A "trackball" **(I)** places the dot or range markers (calipers) anywhere on the display. In general, this must be preceded by activating the measurement mode or annotation mode. To facilitate the review by others, the appropriate body marker **(L)** should be selected and the position of the transducer marked by the trackball **(I)** before the image is printed **(M)**. The remaining functions are less relevant and can be learned by working with the unit.

A Begin with a new patient
B Enter name (ID)
C Menu selection, e.g., abdomen, thyroid gland
D Change of transducer
E Freeze
F Gain
G Depth gain compensation (DGC)
H Image depth/field of view
I Trackball for positioning the dot or range markers
J Measurements
K Annotation
L Body marker
M Image recording

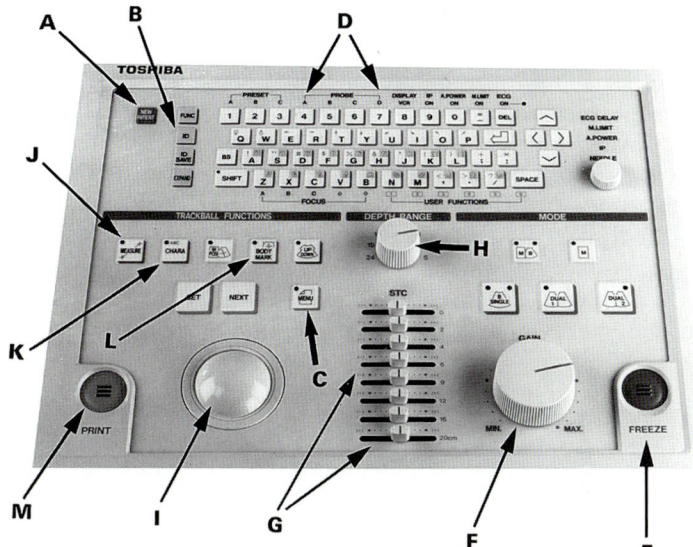

Notes

Sonographic Equipment and Selection of the Appropriate Transducer

Sonographic units used today can be operated with different types of transducers (see below) and are mobile for use in the sonography suite as well as in the intensive care unit or emergency room **(Fig. 8.1)**. The transducers are generally stored on the storage shelf on the right side of the unit.

Precautions should be taken when moving the sonographic unit. Avoid having a dangling transducer cable being caught on a door knob, stretcher, etc., and do not drop a transducer on the floor. Replacing a damaged transducer can be quite expensive! For the same reason, the transducer should never be left unattended on the patient's abdomen when the examination is interrupted, for instance by a phone call. Furthermore, the transducer should be placed upside down to hang with the cable straightened and not pinched or kinked where it enters the transducer (danger of breaking the wires in the cable).

Selection of the appropriate transducer:
Of the many types of transducers only the applications of the three most important ones will be described here.

The linear array transducer emits sound waves parallel to each other and produces a rectangular image. The width of the image and the number of scan lines are constant at all tissue levels **(Fig. 8.2, center)**. An advantage of the linear array transducers is good near-field resolution. They are primarily used with high frequencies (5.0–7.5 MHz) for evaluating soft tissues and the thyroid gland. The disadvantage of these transducers is their large contact surface, leading to artifacts when applied to a curved body contour due to air gaps between the skin and transducer. Furthermore, acoustic shadowing **(45)** as caused by ribs can deteriorate the image **(Fig. 8.2)**. In general, linear array transducers are not suitable for visualizing organs in the thorax or upper abdomen.

A sector transducer produces a fan–like image that is narrow near the transducer and increases in width with deeper penetration **(Fig. 8.2, left)**. This diverging propagation of sound can be achieved by moving the piezo elements mechanically. This is the less expensive solution but has the inherent risk of wear and tear. The electronic version (phased array) is more expensive but has become established primarily in cardiology with frequencies of 2.0–3.0 MHz. The interference of the sound-reflecting ribs can be avoided by applying the transducer to the intercostal space and by taking advantage of the beam's divergency to a 60°- or 90°-sector with increasing depth **(Fig. 8.2)**. The disadvantages of these types of transducer are poor near-field resolution, a decreasing number of scan lines with depth (spatial resolution), and handling difficulties.

Curved or convex array transducers are predominantly used in abdominal sonography with frequencies from 2.5 MHz (obese patients) to 5.0 MHz (slim patients), with the mean value around 3.5–3.75 MHz. As a compromise of both preceding types, it offers a wide near *and* far zone and is handled easier than a sector scan. However, the density of the scan lines decreases with increasing distance from the transducer **(Fig. 8.2, right)**. When scanning the upper abdominal organs, the transducer has to be carefully manipulated to avoid acoustic shadowing **(45)** of the lower ribs.

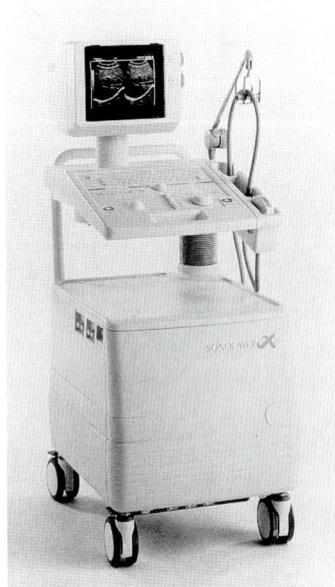

Fig. 8.1

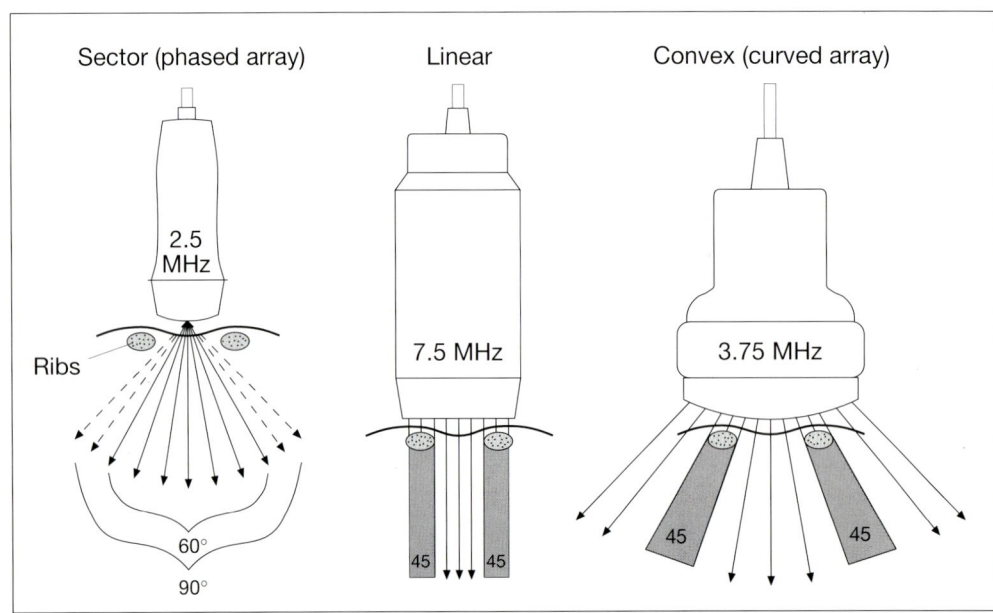

Fig. 8.2

Artifacts

Cognizance of the physical properties of sound that can mimic pathologic findings is mandatory for the correct interpretation of a sonographic image. The most important artifacts include so-called distal shadowing. An acoustic shadow **(45)** appears as a zone of reduced echogenicity (hypoechoic or anechoic = black) and is found behind a strongly reflecting structure, such as calcium-containing bone. Thus the visualization of soft-tissue structures in the upper abdomen is impeded by overlying ribs, and those of the lower pelvis by the pubic symphysis. This effect, however, can be exploited to reveal calcific gallstones **(49) (Fig. 9.2)**, renal stones **(49) (Figs. 42.1, 42.2)**, and atherosclerotic plaques **(49) (Fig. 9.3)**. Similar shadowing can be caused by air in the lungs or intestinal tract. Evaluating structures behind air-containing bowel loops **(46)** is often precluded by acoustic shadowing **(45)** or echogenic comet-tail artifacts **(Figs. 9.2–9.4)**.

The air artifacts interfere primarily with the evaluation of retroperitoneal organs (pancreas, kidneys, and lymph nodes) behind air-containing stomach or bowel. Adequate visualization, however, is still possible by following the approach described on page 79.

Another characteristic finding is the so-called edge shadowing **(45)** behind cysts **(64)**, principally occurring behind all round cavities that are tangentially hit by sound waves **(Fig. 9.1)**. Edge shadowing is caused by scattering and refraction and can be seen behind the gallbladder **(14)**. **Figure 9.4** requires careful analysis to attribute the acoustic shadow **(45)** to edge shadowing caused by the gallbladder, rather than falsely attribute it to focal sparing of fatty infiltration **(62)** in the liver **(9)**.

Relative distal acoustic enhancement **(70)** is found wherever sound waves travel for some distance through homogeneous fluid. Because of decreased reflection in fluid, the sound waves attenuate less and are of higher amplitude distally in comparison with adjacent sound waves. This produces increased echogenicity that is seen as a bright band **(70)** behind the gallbladder **(14) (Fig. 9.4)**, behind the urinary bladder **(38) (Figs. 10.1–10.3)**, or even behind major vessels such as the aorta **(15) (Fig. 9.3)**. This increased echogenicity is a physical phenomenon unrelated to the true characteristics of the underlying tissue. The acoustic enhancement, however, can be applied to distinguish renal or hepatic cysts from hypoechoic tumors.

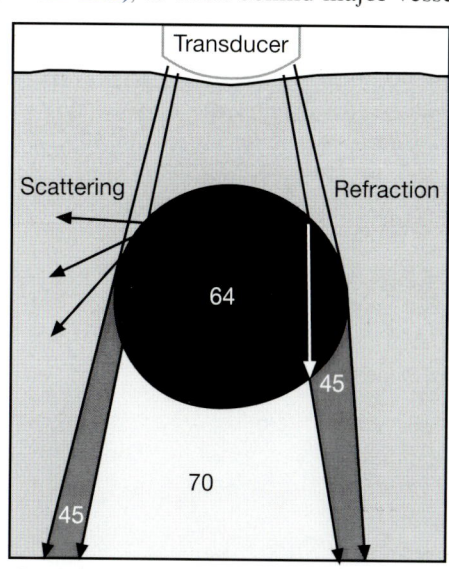

Fig. 9.1

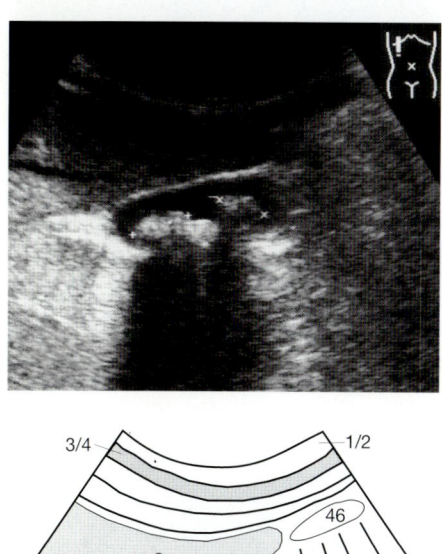
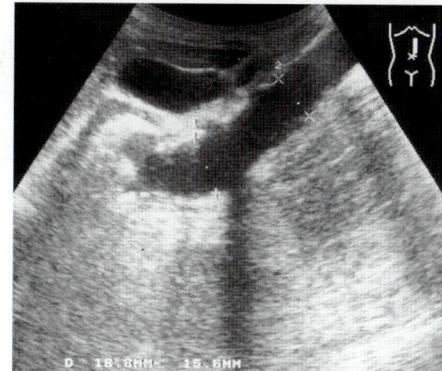
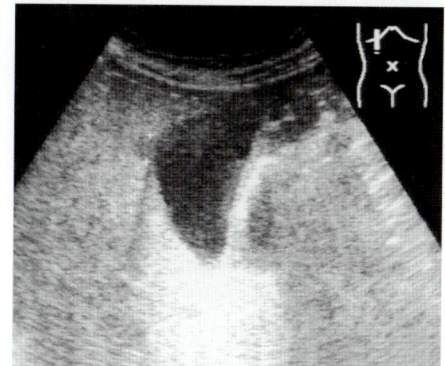
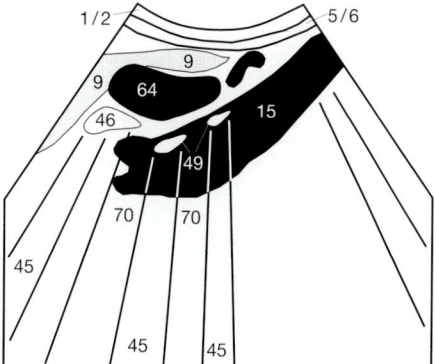
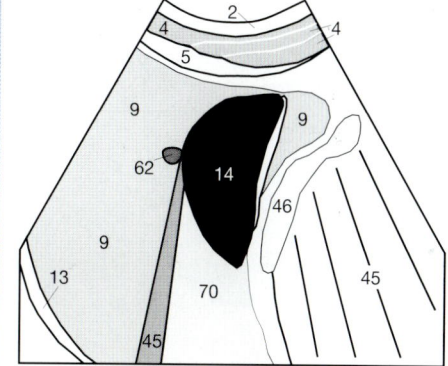

Fig. 9.2 a, b   Fig. 9.3 a, b   Fig. 9.4 a, b

10 Artifacts

Not all echoes that originate at an acoustic interface return to the transducer without further reflection. If several strongly reflecting boundaries are encountered, the sound waves can be reflected back and forth before they eventually return as echo to the transducer. The resultant delay in registering these echoes leads to reverberation echoes (51). These reverberation echoes project as several parallel lines in the anterior aspect (near the transducer) of the urinary bladder (Figs. 10.1 and 10.2) or gallbladder (Fig. 34.3), since the processor calculates the site of the reflection solely from the registered time that has elapsed between emission and recording of the sound pulse by the transducer.

Section-thickness artifacts (51) (Fig. 10.2) are caused when the boundary between the wall of a cyst, gallbladder, or urinary bladder (77) and the containing fluid is not perpendicular to the interrogating sound beam. The echoes within the returning beam include echoes from liquid as well as from solid structures and are averaged by the processor. Consequently, the boundary between solid tissue and fluid is seen as a low echogenic and indistinct structure. Section-thickness artifacts can occasionally mimic sludge or layered material (concrements, blood clots) (52) in the urinary bladder (38) (Fig. 10.3).

Strongly reflecting interfaces can cause a scattered reflection of the echoes, spuriously displacing the acoustic interface laterally as a so-called arch artifact. For instance, the duodenal wall occasionally projects in the lumen of the neighboring gallbladder, or an air-containing bowel loop can be seen within the urinary bladder (Fig. 57.4). Finally, mirror artifacts are primarily produced by the diaphragm and visceral pleura, causing intrahepatic structures to be seen as a mirage on the pulmonary side of the diaphragm (Fig. 27.2b).

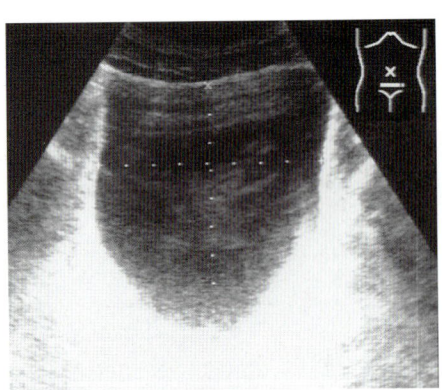

Fig. 10.1 a

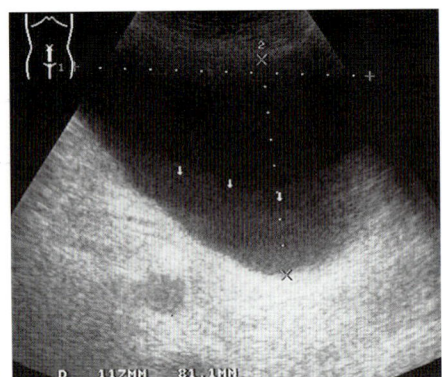

Fig. 10.2 a

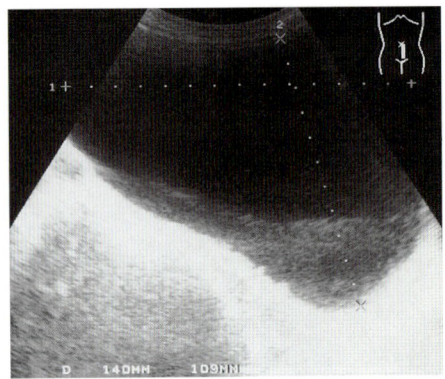

Fig. 10.3 a

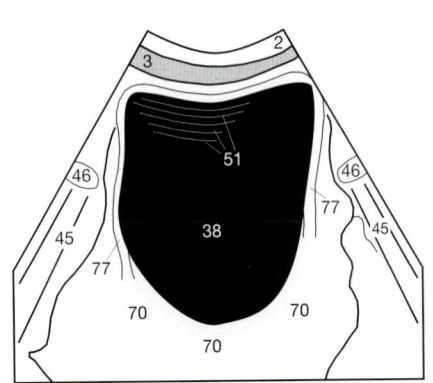

Fig. 10.1 b

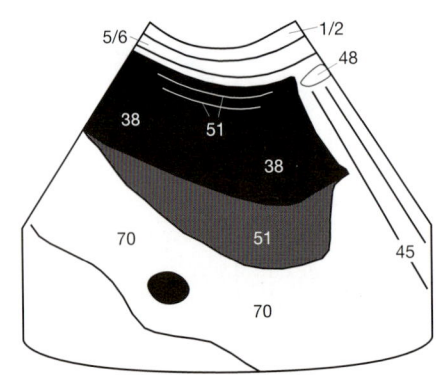

Fig. 10.2 b

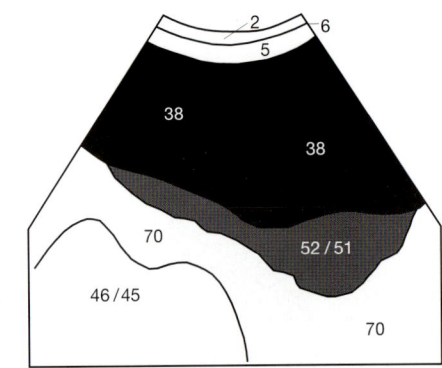

Fig. 10.3 b

1 Sagittal Overview — Upper Retroperitoneum

Did you already mark a cone coffee filter with the location of the structures visualized on sagittal sections, as described on page 4? If not, please do so and compare your drawings with the results on page 78. Only thereafter should you proceed.

The transducer should be perpendicularly placed on the epigastric region along the linea alba and the sound beam swept through the upper abdomen in a fan–like fashion **(Fig. 11.1)**. For the time being, it should suffice to memorize the appearance of the normal anatomy. With the transducer inclined to the patient's *right* side **(Fig. 11.2)**, aorta **(15)**, celiac axis **(32)**, and superior mesenteric artery (SMA) **(17)** are found paravertebrally on the left and dorsal to the liver **(9)**. Normally, all major vessels are hypoechoic (dark) or anechoic (black).

The image displays the superiorly located diaphragm **(13)** on the left and the more inferiorly located pancreas **(33)** and confluens **(12)** of the portal vein **(11)** on the right. The hypoechoic extensions of the diaphragm (the diaphragmatic crura) **(13)** and the gastroesophageal junction **(34)** are shown anterior to the aorta and immediately below the diaphragm. It is important to note where the left renal vein **(25)** crosses the aorta to reach the right-sided inferior vena cava. It travels through the narrow space between aorta and SMA, immediately caudal to the aortic origin of the SMA. If not well demonstrated, the uninitiated examiner might mistake this vessel for a hypoechoic lymph node. Comparison with the transverse section at the same level clarifies this finding further **(Fig. 18.3)**.

Now the transducer is inclined to the patient's *left* side **(Fig. 11.3)** for the visualization of the right paravertebrally situated inferior vena cava **(16)**, including its continuation into the right atrium. At the same level, the hepatic veins **(10)** can be distinguished from intrahepatic branches of the portal vein **(11)**.

The presence of air prevents evaluation of the lungs **(47)**. The diameter of the inferior vena cava should not exceed 2.0 cm or, in young athletes, 2.5 cm. The maximum diameter of 2.5 cm also applies to the aortic lumen at this level. The luminal diameter is always measured perpendicular to the vessel's longitudinal axis. The $d_{AO} = 1.8$ cm and $d_{VC} = 2.3$ cm in the cases illustrated here **(Figs. 11.2, 11.3)** are within the normal range.

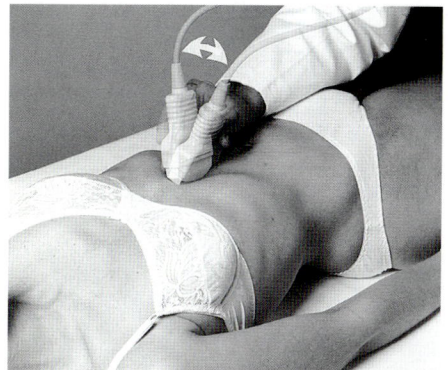

Fig. 11.1

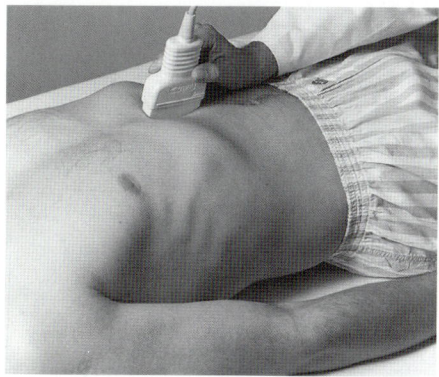

Fig. 11.2 a

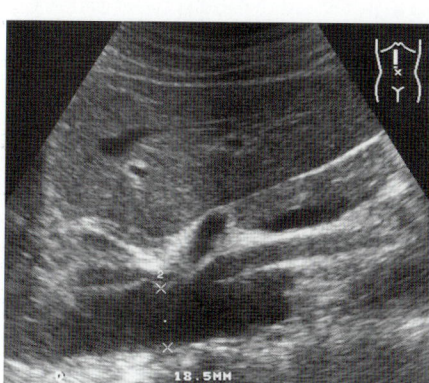

Fig. 11.2 b

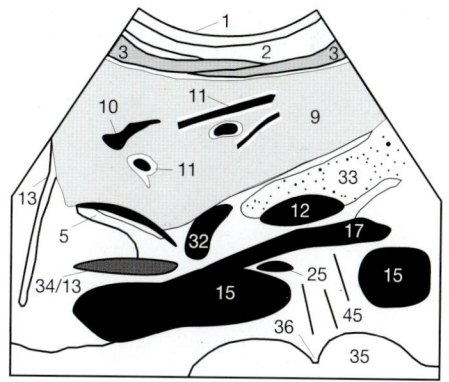

Fig. 11.2 c

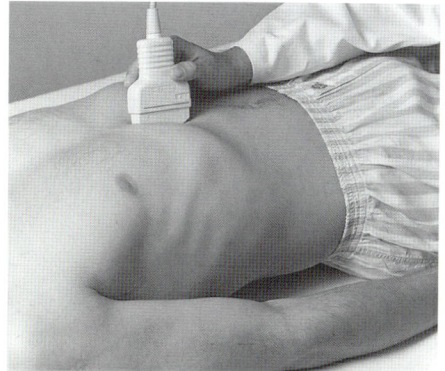

Fig. 11.3 a

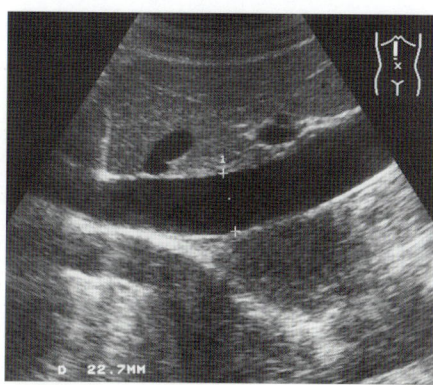

Fig. 11.3 b

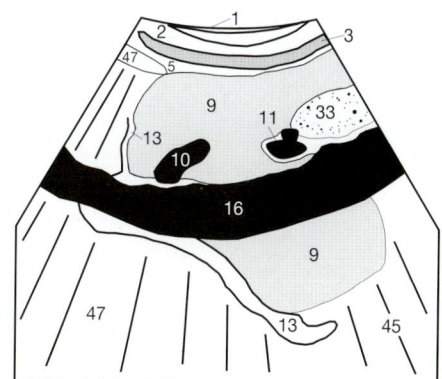

Fig. 11.3 c

1 Sagittal Overview — Lower Peritoneum in Oblique Sections: Normal Findings

After the upper retroperitoneum has been scanned, the transducer is moved inferiorly (arrow) along the aorta and inferior vena cava **(Fig. 12.1 a)**. While the transducer is being moved, the vascular lumina should be visualized and evaluated and the perivascular spaces searched for space-occupying lesions. Preferably, the examination should be biplanar by adding transverse sections (see pp. 17 and 18). Enlarged lymph nodes are characteristically visualized as ovoid to lobulated space-occupying lesions with a hypoechoic pattern (see pp. 14 and 21). Distal to the aortic bifurcation, the branching iliac vessels are delineated and evaluated in two planes by sweeping the sound beam parallel **(Fig. 12.1 b)** and perpendicular **(Fig. 12.1 c)** to the longitudinal vascular axis.

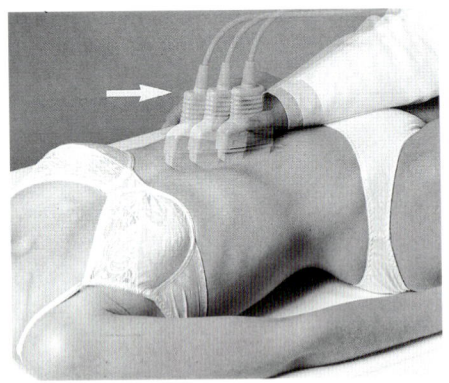
Fig. 12.1 a

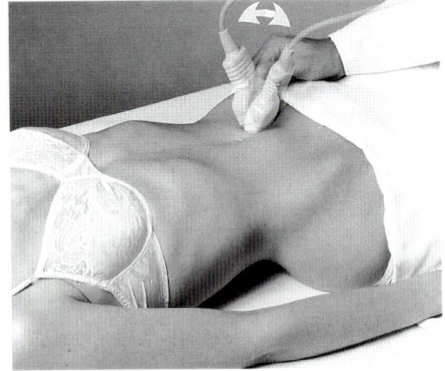
Fig. 12.1 b

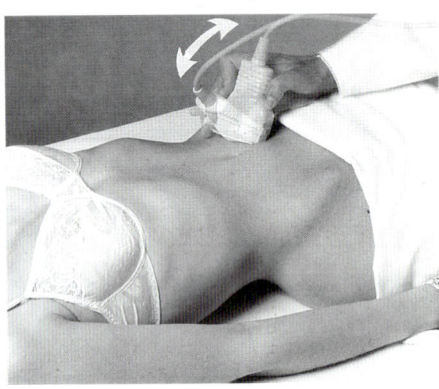
Fig. 12.1 c

The confluence of the external **(22)** and internal **(23)** iliac veins is a frequent site for regional nodal enlargement **(Fig. 12.2)**. The iliac artery **(21)** is anterior (i.e., superior on the image) to the vein. In unclear cases, the compression test can differentiate these structures, with the vein as a low pressure system showing easy compressibility. On transverse section **(Fig. 12.3)**, the iliac vessels can be easily distinguished from hypoechoic fluid-filled intestinal loops **(46)** by the peristalsis of the intestinal wall.

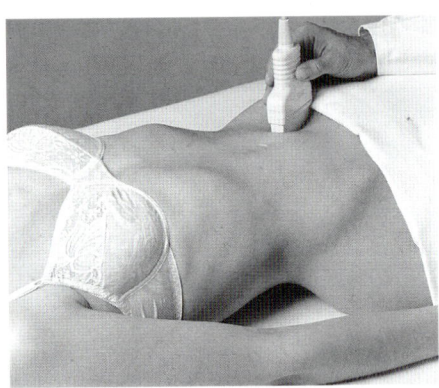
Fig. 12.2 a

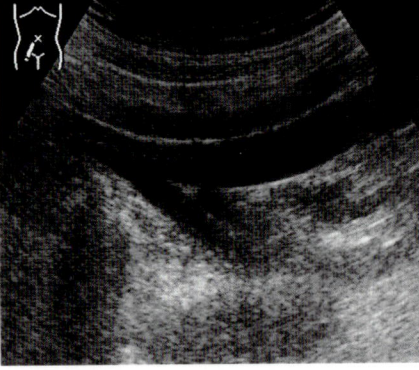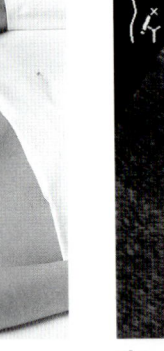
Fig. 12.2 b

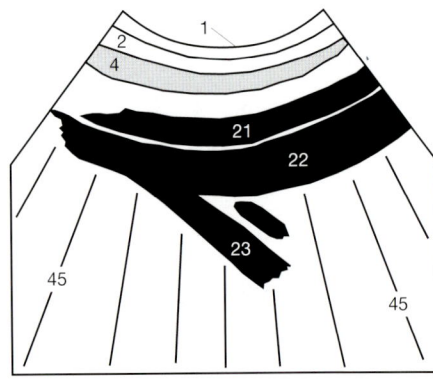
Fig. 12.2 c

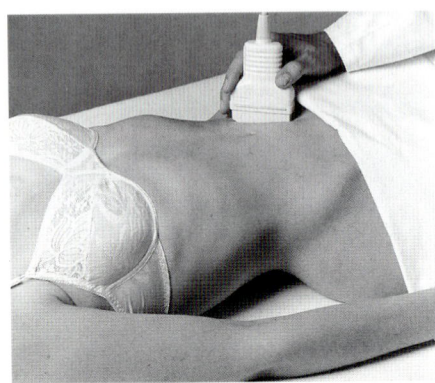
Fig. 12.3 a

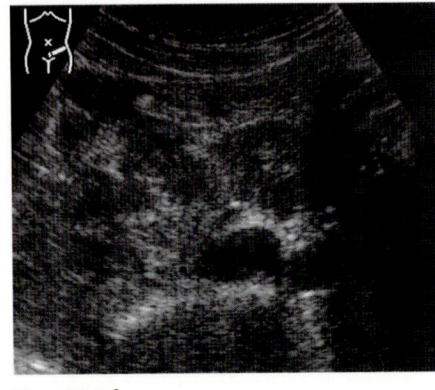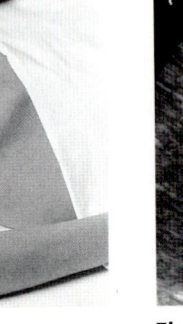
Fig. 12.3 b

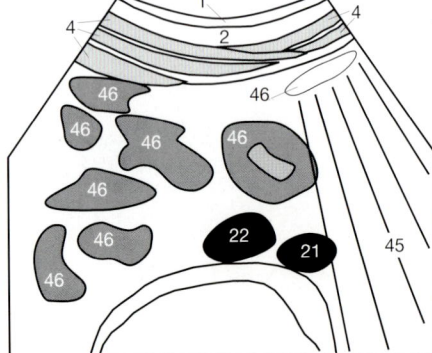
Fig. 12.3 c

1 Sagittal Overview — Aortic Ectasia and Aneurysms

Localized dilatations of the vascular lumen are generally caused by atherosclerotic lesions and local weakening of the arterial wall. They are rarely posttraumatic. A dilatation of up to 3 cm is referred to as ectasia and can be found in addition to an aneurysm **(Fig. 13.1)**.

The dilatation can be fusiform or saccular. It can be complicated by dissection of the arterial wall (dissecting aneurysm) or circumferential intraluminal clot formation **(52)** with possible peripheral emboli. Risk factors for rupture of an aortic aneurysm are a diameter of greater than 6 cm, an excentric lumen, and diverticulum–like bulging of the aortic wall. As general rule, the risk of a rupture increases with the size of the aneurysm and patients with an aortic aneurysm exceeding 5 cm in diameter should be assessed clinically for surgical repair.

If an aneurysm is detected, the sonographic examination should report its maximal length **(Fig. 13.2)** and diameter **(Fig. 13.3)** as well as any detected thrombi **(52)** and possible involvement of the renal and iliac arteries. Though most aortic aneurysms are infrarenal, their exact extent should be established before surgical intervention. Any aneurysmal bleeding primarily occurs into the retroperitoneum but can extend into the peritoneal cavity in the presence of high pressure.

Checklist Aortic Aneurysm:
- Normal lumen:
  suprarenal < 2.5 cm
- Ectasia: 2.5–3.0 cm
- Aneurysm: > 3 cm
- Risk of rupture increased by:
  progressing dilatation
  diameter > 6 cm
  excentric lumen
  saccular dilatation
  (instead of fusiform dilatation)

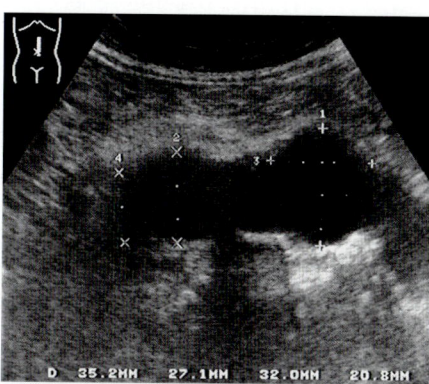
Fig. 13.1 a

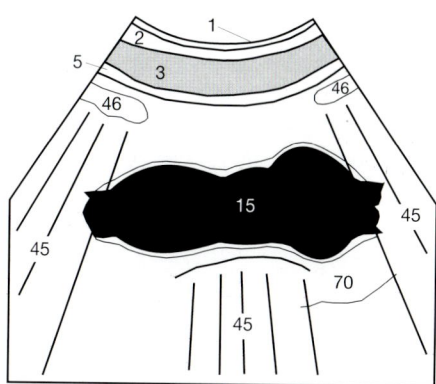
Fig. 13.1 b

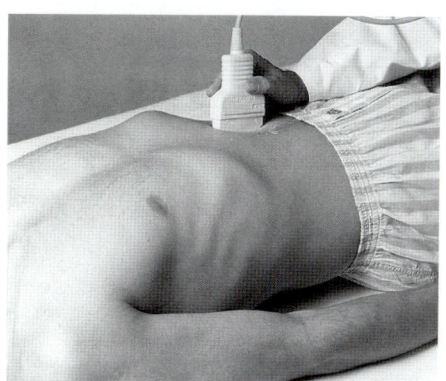
Fig. 13.2 a

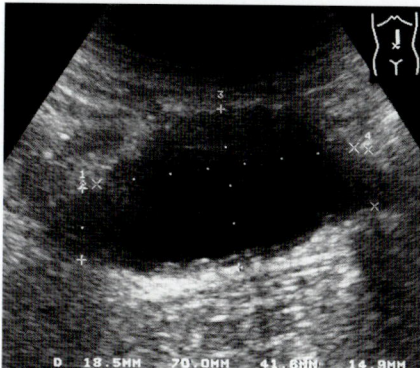
Fig. 13.2 b

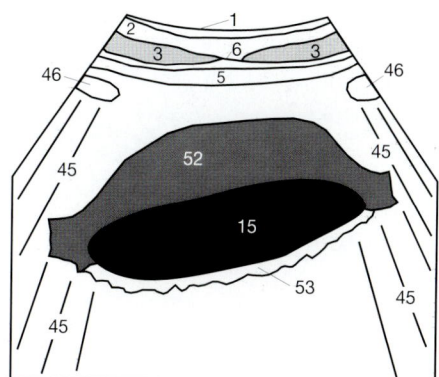
Fig. 13.2 c

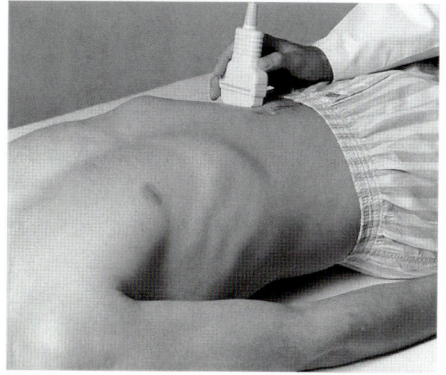
Fig. 13.3 a

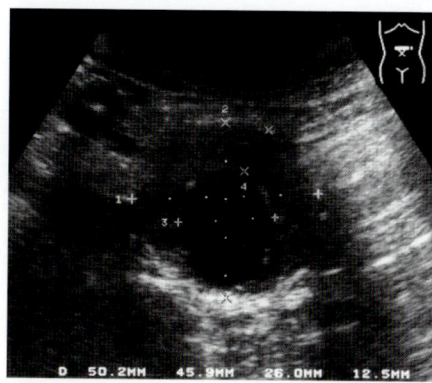
Fig. 13.3 b

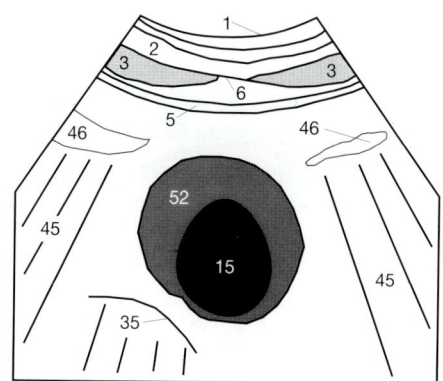
Fig. 13.3 c

1 Sagittal Overview — Retroperitoneum: Lymph Nodes

Lymph nodes **(55)** are generally hypoechoic and must be differentiated from fluid-filled bowel loops **(46)** by absent peristalsis and from veins by lack of compressibility. Computerized tomography (CT) is superior in evaluating thrombosed veins (non-compressible) or markedly obese patients, but sonography is advantageous in very thin or cachectic patients. Enlarged lymph nodes can be found with inflammation, malignant lymphoma (Hodgkin disease or non-Hodgkin lymphoma), and metastatic deposits.

The normal size of abdominal lymph nodes is given as 7–10 mm. Larger and still normal lymph nodes measuring up to 20 mm in longitudinal diameter can be found in the inguinal region and along the distal external iliac artery **(21)** **(Fig. 14.3)**. Important for all enlarged lymph nodes are follow-up examinations to determine any possible progression or regression—for instance, for the evaluation of chemotherapy. Furthermore, any possible hepatomegaly or splenomegaly should be documented and quantified.

Lymph nodes with inflammatory changes maintain their ovoid shape, have a distinct border, and exhibit two layers with a centrally increased echogenicity at the hilum (hilar fat sign) and peripheral liver–like echogenicity. Inflammatory lymph nodes can often be encountered along the hepatoduodenal ligament **(Fig. 24.3)** accompanying viral hepatitis, cholangitis, or pancreatitis **(Fig. 19.3)**.

In contrast, metastatic lymph nodes are more round than oval, frequently of heterogeneous echogenicity, and indistinct in outline. They also have the tendency to form aggregates. The site of the primary tumor can be deduced from the known lymphatic pathways; para-aortic lymphadenopathy in young men, for instance, suggests a testicular tumor.

Enlarged lymph nodes as manifestation of malignant lymphoma generally exhibit an ovoid form, smooth margins, and more pronounced hypoechogenicity than found in inflammatory or metastatic lymph nodes. In one third of cases, the spleen shows concomitant focal or diffuse involvement **(Fig. 48.1)**. Predominant involvement of the mesenteric lymph nodes **(55)** **(Figs. 14.1, 14.2)** suggests a non-Hodgkin lymphoma and not Hodgkin disease, which has a predilection for thoracic and retroperitoneal lymph nodes. Malignant lymphomas indent or displace adjacent vessels **(Fig. 14.2)** but respect the vascular wall and do not invade adjacent organs (see also p. 21).

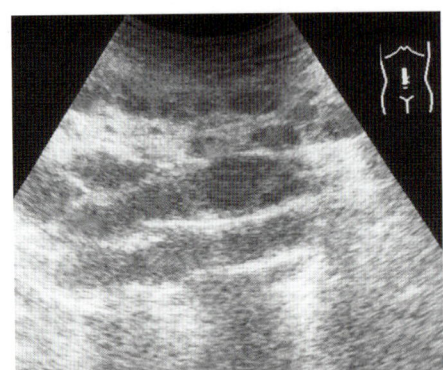

Fig. 14.1 a

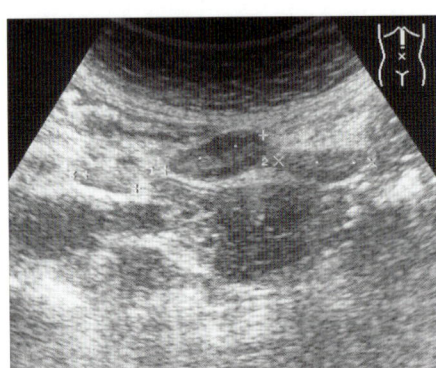

Fig. 14.2 a

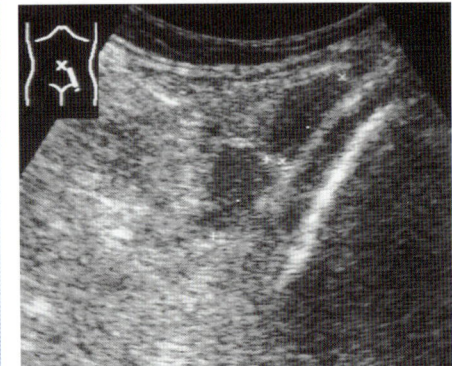

Fig. 14.3 a

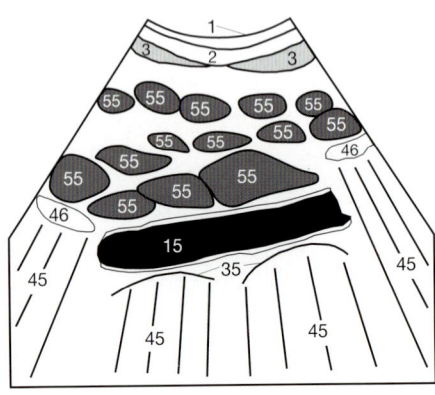

Fig. 14.1 b

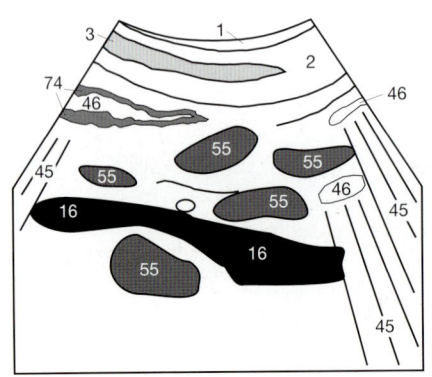

Fig. 14.2 b

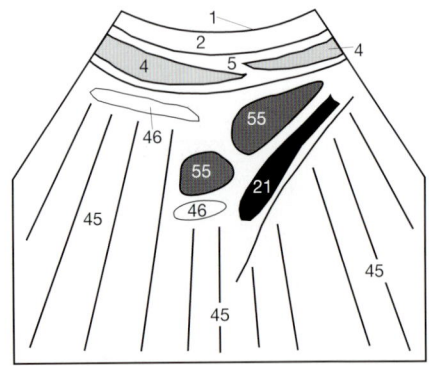

Fig. 14.3 b

1 Sagittal Overview — Retroperitoneum: Other Clinical Cases

The systematic evaluation of the retroperitoneum should delineate and document all abnormalities of the major vessels. Atherosclerotic plaques (49) along the aorta can be seen directly by their echogenicity or indirectly by their acoustic shadowing (45) (Fig. 15.1).

The inferior vena cava (16) should be evaluated for a dilatation exceeding 2 cm (or 2.5 cm in young athletes), which would suggest a venous congestion as manifestation of a right cardiac insufficiency (Fig. 15.2). The measurements are obtained perpendicular to the longitudinal vascular axis (!) and should not accidentally encompass the hepatic veins (10), which enter the inferior vena cava subdiaphragmatically (Fig. 15.2). In questionable cases, the luminal diameter of the inferior vena cava is observed during forced maximal inspiration, which can be achieved by asking the patient to take a deep breath with the mouth open. The transmitted sudden increase in intrapleural negative pressure causes a brief collapse of the subdiaphragmatic portion of the normal inferior vena cava, with the lumen being reduced to a third or less of its diameter during quiet respiration. With fluid overload of the right cardiac atrium, the cava does not collapse during forced inspiration. During the thoracic movement of this maneuver, it can be difficult to stay with the same sonographic section of the inferior vena cava. For further clarification, the luminal diameter of the hepatic vein should be assessed in the right subcostal oblique section (see p. 25). Do you remember why in **Figure 15.2** the hepatic parenchyma appears more echogenic dorsal to the distended inferior vena cava than anterior to it? If not, return to page 9 and name this phenomenon.

When visualizing the distal iliac vessels (Fig. 15.3) following an inguinal vascular puncture, a hematoma (50) can occasionally be encountered adjacent to the iliac artery (21) or vein (22). If blood flows into this perivascular space through a connection with the arterial lumen, a false aneurysm (aneurysma spurium) is present. This type of aneurysm differs from a true aneurysm (aneurysma verum), which represents luminal widening of all mural layers and is not caused by a complete mural tear (Fig. 15.3). Old inguinal hematomas must be differentiated from psoas abscesses and synovial cysts arising from the hip joint, and, when extending into the lower pelvis, from lymphoceles, large ovarian cysts, and metastatic lymph nodes with central necrosis (57).

> **Checklist Right cardiac Insufficiency:**
> - Dilatation of the inferor vena cava — to > 2.0 cm (2.5 cm in trained athletes)
> - Dilated hepatic veins — > 6 mm in the hepatic periphery
> - Absent caval collapse with forced inspiration
> - Possible pleural effusion, initially almost always on the right

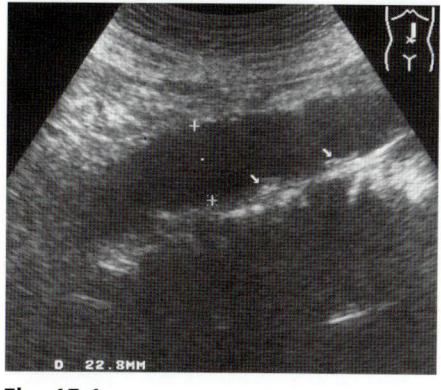

Fig. 15.1 a

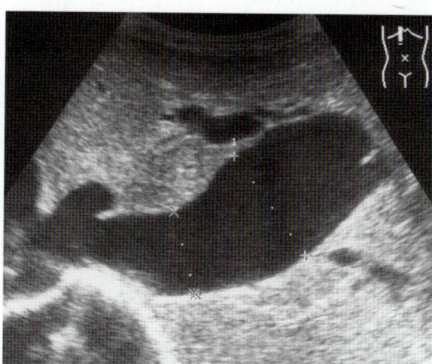

Fig. 15.2 a

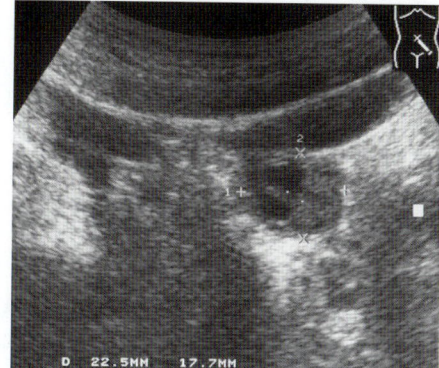

Fig. 15.3 a

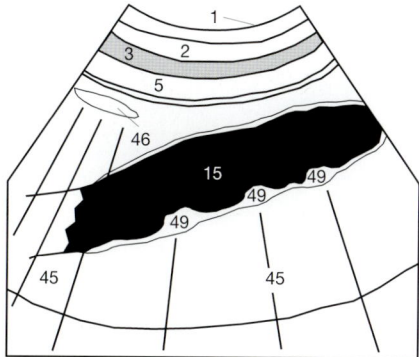

Fig. 15.1 b

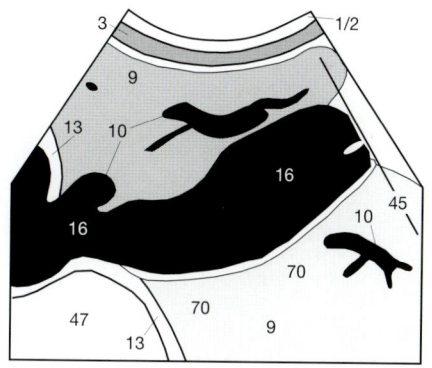

Fig. 15.2 b

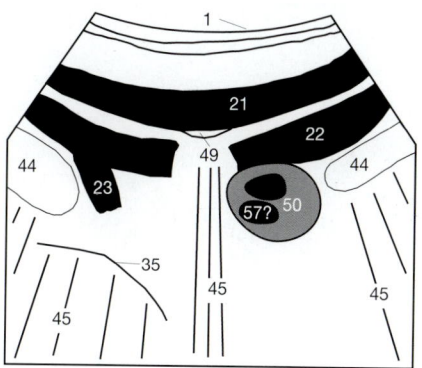

Fig. 15.3 b

1 Sagittal Overview — Quiz for Self-Assessment

Before turning to the material of the following section, the following questions should be answered to test whether the goal of the first lesson has been achieved. The answers to questions 1 to 6 can be found on the preceding pages. The answers to the figure of question 7 can be looked up on page 76 *after* the individual questions listed in the text have been addressed.

1 Which side of the body corresponds to the left side of the image? Superior or inferior? Where is anterior in the image, and where are the posterior structures?

2 What is the luminal diameter of the inferior vena cava and abdominal aorta (upper limits of normal) in cm? How is aortic ectasia defined and from what luminal width in cm is it called an aneurysm?

3 What procedure can be added when the luminal diameter of the inferior vena cava is borderline and a right cardiac insufficiency must be excluded?

4 What vessel crosses between the aorta and SMA to the contralateral side on the sagittal image and can mimic a hypoechoic lymphoma? At what level is this vascular crossing?

5 What is the maximum longitudinal diameter of retroperitoneal lymph nodes that can still be called normal? What is the value of follow-up examinations for the evaluation of visualized lymph nodes?

6 Look at the three transducers shown. Which transducer is used for which body region? What is the rationale? What frequency (in MHz) belongs to each transducer? Write the answer below each transducer.

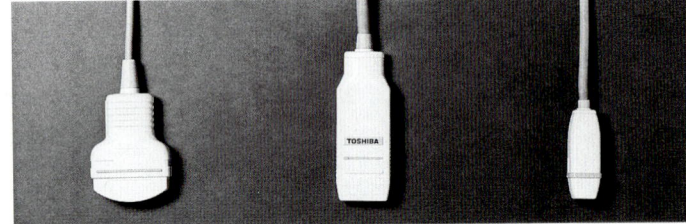

Fig. 16.1

7 Review this image step by step. What is the imaging plane? Which organs are shown? Name all structures, if possible. How does the image differ from a normal image? Try to give a differential diagnosis.

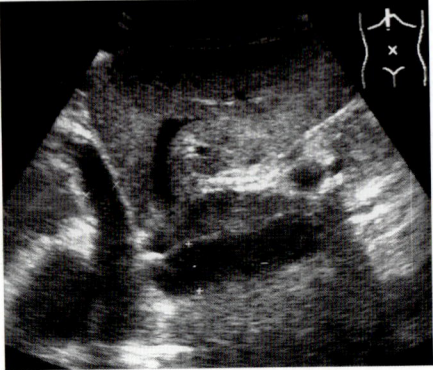

Fig. 16.2

2 Axial Overview — Upper Abdomen: Basic Anatomy

Working through the following pages should be preceded by a review of the sonographic sections obtained in the transverse plane. Where is the liver on a correctly oriented sonographic transverse section? Right or left? If you cannot answer this with certainty you should consult page 4 and recapitulate the intricate anatomic relationship of the organs as seen on transverse images by means of a cone coffee filter (the solution is found on p. 78).

The transducer is turned 90° and placed horizontally on the upper abdomen. With the patient taking a deep breath and holding it, the upper abdomen is systematically reviewed while the transducer is moved slowly and steadily in craniocaudal direction (Fig. 17.1). By following the course of the vessels, they can be easily identified.

On these transverse sections, the examiner is confronted with a multitude of arteries, veins, biliary ducts, and lymph nodes, all confined to a small space and demanding differentiation from each other (all vessels are hypoechoic, but so are lymph nodes). Do you remember where the left renal vein crosses to the contralateral right side, or whether the right renal artery is anterior or posterior to the inferior vena cava to the right kidney? Refresh your basic anatomic knowledge by writing the names of all the numbered structures in Figure 17.2 and 17.3 below both figures and thereafter unfold the back cover page to compare your list with the key. Review again the topography of pancreas, duodenum, and spleen in relation to the major abdominal vessels as illustrated in Figure 17.3. To make the review easy, the three most important transverse sections of the upper abdomen are described and illustrated on the next page.

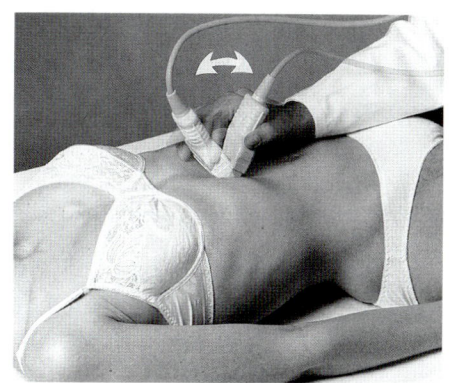

Fig. 17.1

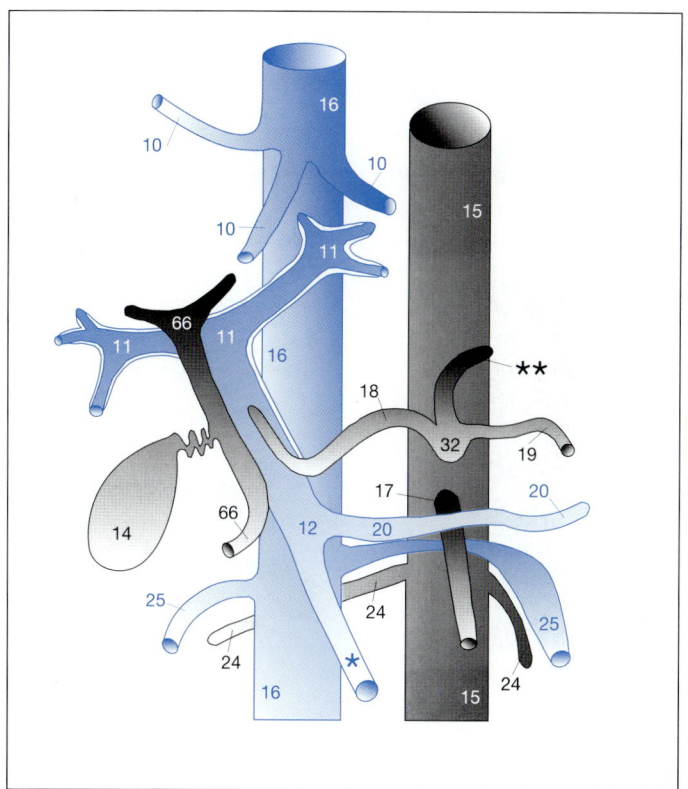

Fig. 17.2

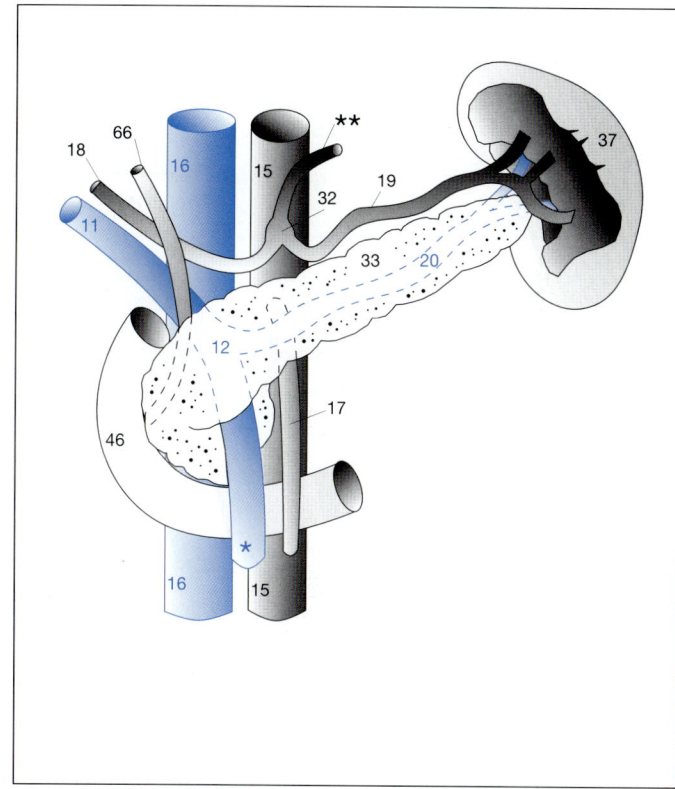

Fig. 17.3

Notes

2 Axial Overview — Upper Abdomen: Normal Findings

First, the patient has to take a deep breath and hold it, so that the inferiorly displaced liver can serve as an acoustic window for the pancreas and lesser sac, including the major vessels traversing it (see p. 79). Skin **(1)**, subcutaneous fat **(2)**, and both rectus muscles **(3)** are directly beneath the transducer. The ligamentum teres **(7)** with the obliterated umbilical vein can be delineated posterior to the linea alba **(6)**, particularly in obese patients. The lesser sac is seen as a small cleft posterior to the liver **(9)** and, further posterior to it, the pancreas **(33)**. The tail of the pancreas is often obscured by air shadows **(45)** arising from the stomach **(26)**. The splenic vein **(20)** always runs directly along the posterior border of the pancreas. The renal vein **(25)**, however, is more posterior between the SMA **(17)** and aorta **(15)**, and is only imaged on more caudal sections **(Fig. 18.3)**. A more cranial transverse section **(Fig. 18.1)** visualizes the celiac axis **(32)** together with the hepatic **(18)** and splenic **(19)** arteries. The gastric artery is generally not visualized. The origin of the SMA **(17)** is more caudal by about 1–2 cm **(Fig. 18.2)**, as clearly illustrated on the sagittal images **(Fig. 11.2)**. It should be noted that the display inverts the position of the organs (which are shown as if viewed from the patient's feet). The inferior vena cava **(16)**, seen as an ovoid structure, is on the *left* side of the image, and the aorta **(15)**, seen as a round structure, is on the *right* side anterior to the spine **(35)**. The head of the pancreas **(33)** characteristically surrounds the confluens **(12)** of the portal vein **(11)**, which is frequently obscured by duodenal air **(46)** in the region of the lesser omentum.

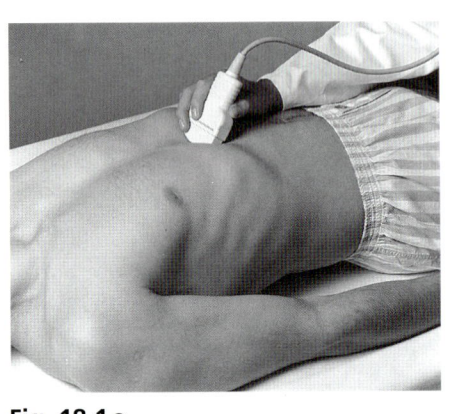
Fig. 18.1 a

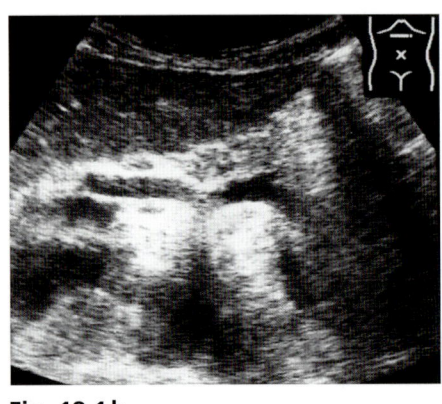
Fig. 18.1 b

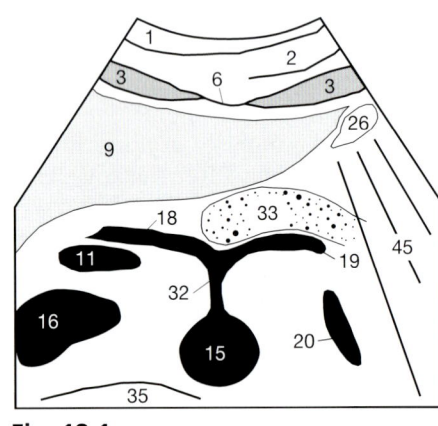
Fig. 18.1 c

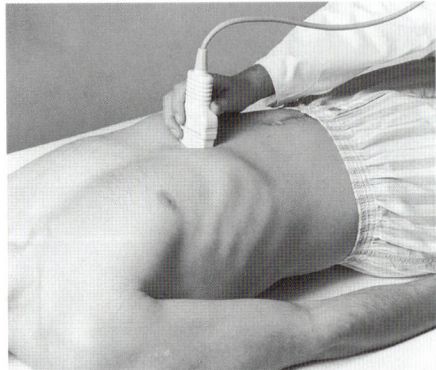
Fig. 18.2 a

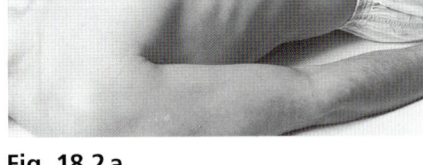

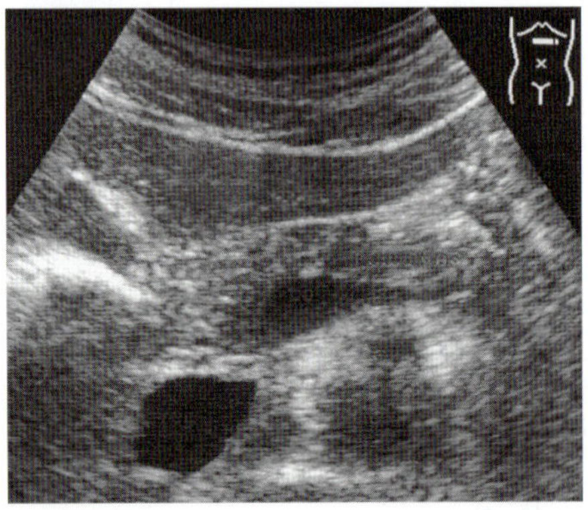

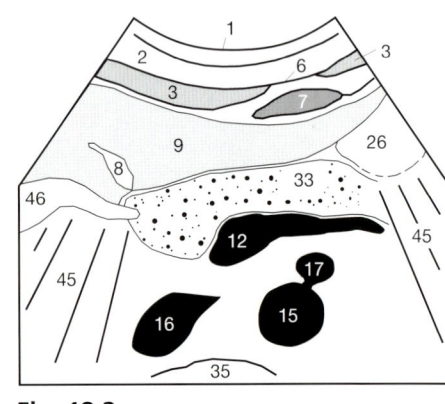
Fig. 18.2 b — Fig. 18.2 c

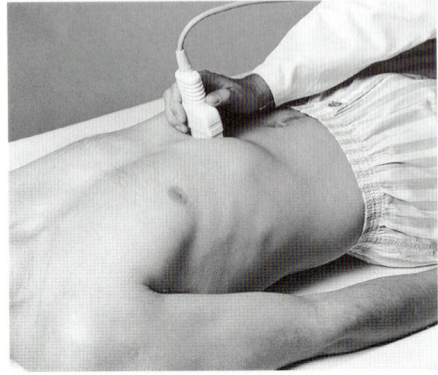
Fig. 18.3 a

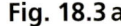

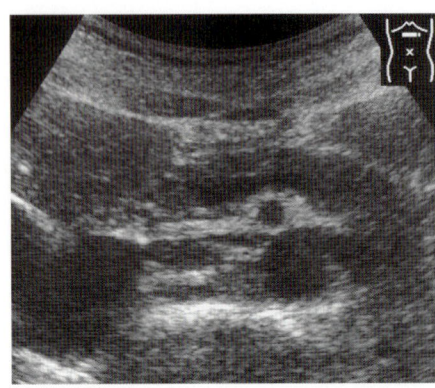
Fig. 18.3 b

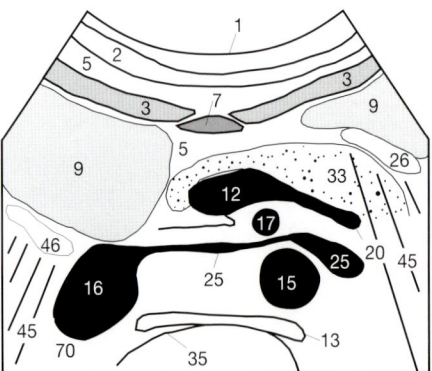
Fig. 18.3 c

2 Axial Overview — Upper Abdomen: Pancreatitis

The echogenicity of the pancreas changes with increasing age. In young and slim patients, the parenchyma is hypoechoic in comparison with the surrounding tissue, including the hepatic parenchyma. The deposition of fat in the pancreas (pancreatic lipomatosis) can be found in older or obese patients and causes the parenchyma to increase its echogenicity, leading to a hyperechoic, i.e., brighter, appearance of the pancreas. The normal anteroposterior diameters of the pancreas are somewhat variable and should be less than 3 cm for its head and less than 2.5 cm for its body and tail. The causes of pancreatitis include biliary obstruction (cholestasis) secondary to a stone lodged in the distal common bile duct (biliary pancreatitis), increased viscosity of the bile secondary to parenteral nutrition and, above all, alcoholism (alcohol pancreatitis), which is, among others, related to protein plugs obstructing the small pancreatic duct.

Acute pancreatitis of the first degree can initially be devoid of any sonomorphologic changes. The edema found in more advanced stages causes marked hypoechogenicity, increased thickness, and indistinctness of the pancreas (33). Chronic pancreatitis is characterized by a heterogeneous fibrosis (Fig. 19.1), calcific deposits (53), and an undulated, irregular outline of the pancreas (Figs. 19.1, 19.2). Moreover, a beaded or irregular dilatation of the pancreatic duct (75) can occur (Fig. 19.2). The normal pancreatic duct is smoothly outlined and measures up to 2 mm in diameter. Inflammatory lymph nodes (Fig. 19.3) in the vicinity of the pancreas, for instance anterior to the portal vein (11), can accompany pancreatitis.

The real contribution of sonography is not the early diagnosis of acute pancreatitis. This can be better achieved by laboratory tests or CT, particularly in view of the markedly increased bowel gas encountered with an acutely inflamed pancreas and interfering with sonographic imaging. Sonography has the role of excluding other diagnostic possibilities, such as cholecystitis, choledocholithiasis, and aortic aneurysm. Furthermore, sonography can be used to follow the pancreatitis and to detect its complications, such as inflammatory infiltration of the neighboring duodenal or gastric wall (46, 26) and thrombophlebitis of the adjacent splenic vein (20). It might be necessary to add color Doppler sonography of the splenic vein if the conventional sonographic evaluation of the spleen is normal. Moreover, necrotic paths in the retroperitoneum (grade II acute pancreatitis) and the development of pseudocysts should be discovered early, so that surgical intervention or puncture under sonographic or CT guidance can be carried out, if indicated, without undue delay. The inflammation does not always involve the entire pancreas, and segmental and "channel" pancreatitis confined to certain segments of the pancreas or along its duodenal surface can be encountered. These manifestations cannot always be reliably differentiated from other localized space-occupying processes, such as a carcinoma.

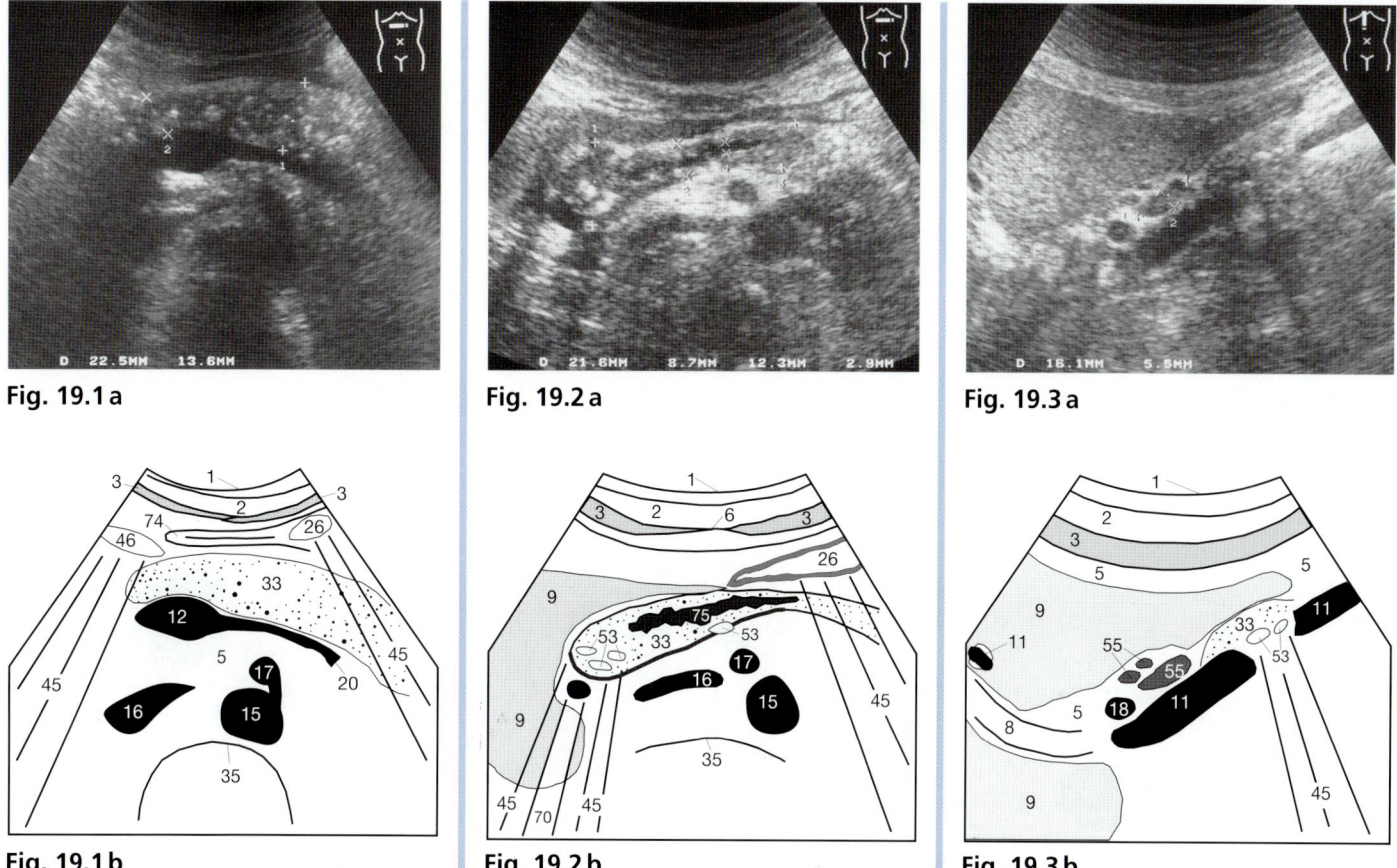

Fig. 19.1 a Fig. 19.2 a Fig. 19.3 a

Fig. 19.1 b Fig. 19.2 b Fig. 19.3 b

2 Axial Overview

Pancreas: Additional Cases

Looking at the normal echogenicity of the pancreas (33) on longitudinal (Fig. 11.2) or transverse sections (Fig. 18.3) reveals no appreciable difference in comparison with the echogenicity of the liver. With increasing age or obesity, the echogenicity increases as a manifestation of pancreatic lipomatosis (Fig. 20.1). This accentuates the contrast between pancreas and hypoechoic splenic vein (20).

Tumors of the pancreas (54) are generally more hypoechoic than the remaining pancreas and are sometimes not easily differentiated from adjacent bowel loops (by peristalsis) or space-occupying lesions arising from peripancreatic lymph nodes (see p. 21). Pancreatic carcinomas have a poor prognosis and remain clinically silent for a long time. They are often only detected after they have metastasized, when they compress the common bile duct, or after they have led to an otherwise unexplained weight loss. Early retroperitoneal extension, nodal or hepatic metastases, and/or peritoneal carcinomatosis are responsible for the poor 5-year survival rate, which is far below 10%.

Endocrine pancreatic tumors are generally small at the time of diagnosis because of their systemic hormonal effects and, as all small pancreatic tumors, are best visualized by endosonography (Fig. 20.3). An annular transducer at the tip of an endoscope is positioned into the stomach or through the pylorus into the duodenum, surrounded by a water-filled balloon for acoustic coupling with the gastric or duodenal wall.

Because of the short penetration needed to reach the target structure, a high frequency (5–10 MHz) can be selected, resulting in improved resolution. The same principle is used in transesophageal echocardiography that also has, because of the use of high-frequency transducers, a markedly improved image quality in comparison with transthoracic echocardiography.

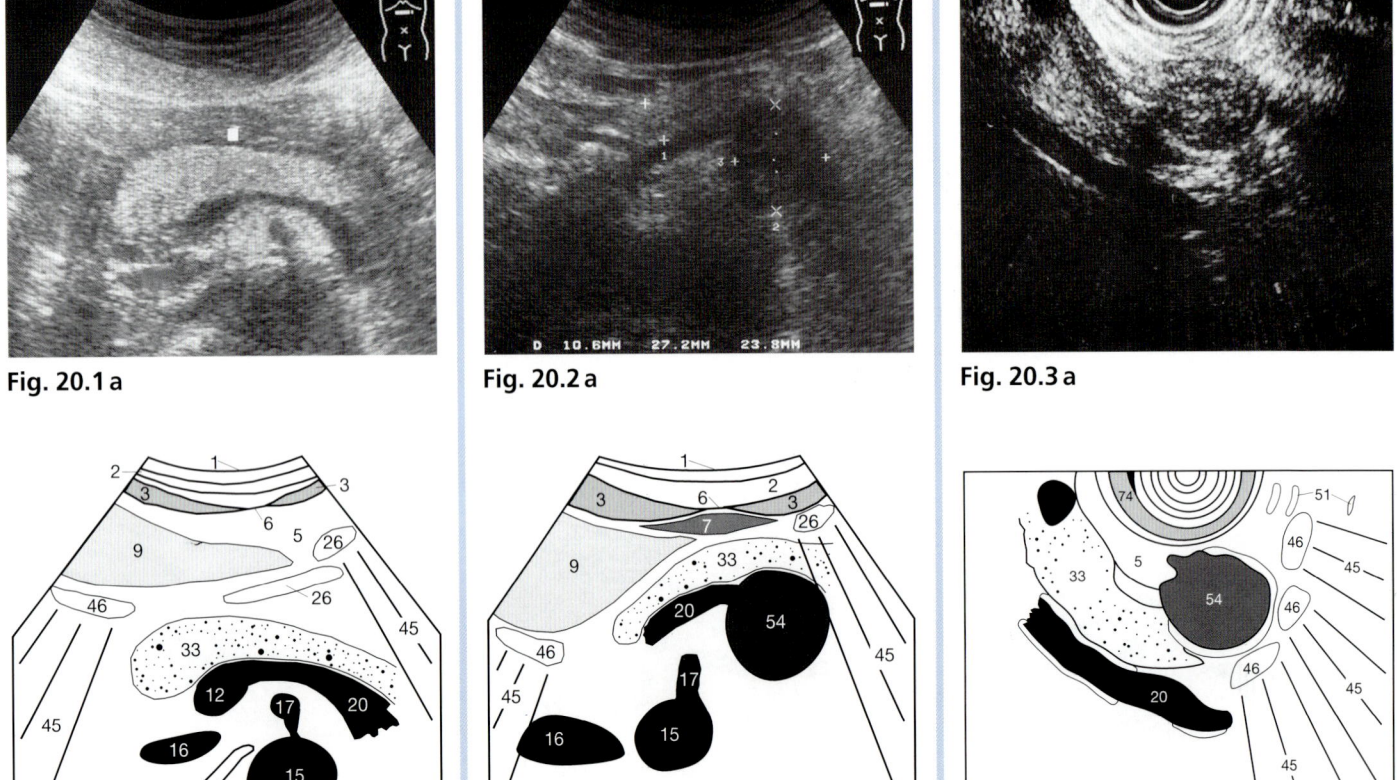

Fig. 20.1 a Fig. 20.2 a Fig. 20.3 a

Fig. 20.1 b Fig. 20.2 b Fig. 20.3 b

2 Axial Overview — Upper Abdomen: Lymph Nodes

The criteria distinguishing inflammatory lymph nodes from metastatic and lymphomatous lymph nodes were already discussed on page 14. Depending on the incidence angle, the upper abdominal vessels **(15, 16)** can be visualized as ovoid structures on transverse sections and must be distinguished from pathologic lymph nodes **(Figs. 21.1, 21.2)**. Familiarity with the normal vascular anatomy is therefore fundamental. Very hypoechoic lymph nodes that lack an echogenic hilus and displace, but do not invade, adjacent veins are suggestive of the presence of a lymphoma, such as chronic lymphatic leukemia **(Fig. 21.2)**. The pathologic lymph node shown here is situated directly anterior and to the right of the bifurcation of the celiac axis **(32)** into the common hepatic artery **(18)** and splenic artery **(19)**. The resultant space-occupying effect obliterates the characteristic fluke-like configuration of the celiac axis.

Occasionally, large nodal aggregates **(Fig. 21.1)** can be seen around and virtually "encasing" the retroperitoneal or mesenteric vessels. In such cases, representative lymph nodes are identified and measured to assess any interval growth on subsequent studies. If intra-abdominal or retroperitoneal lymph nodes are encountered, the examination should proceed to measuring the size of the liver and spleen. Both organs must also be searched for heterogeneous infiltrations. Diffuse lymphomatous involvement of the splenic parenchyma does not always translate into sonomorphologic changes, and the infiltrated spleen can appear normal or show only diffuse enlargement **(Fig. 48.1)**. Additional lymphadenopathy must be searched for in the inguinal, axillary and cervical regions. Paralytic fluid-filled intestinal loops are rarely mistaken for lymph nodes. An intestinal diverticulum **(54)** can mimic a tumor or enlarged lymph node, as shown in **Fig. 21.3**. Eliciting peristaltic activity from a paralytic intestinal loop by applying graded compression can clarify the differential diagnosis.

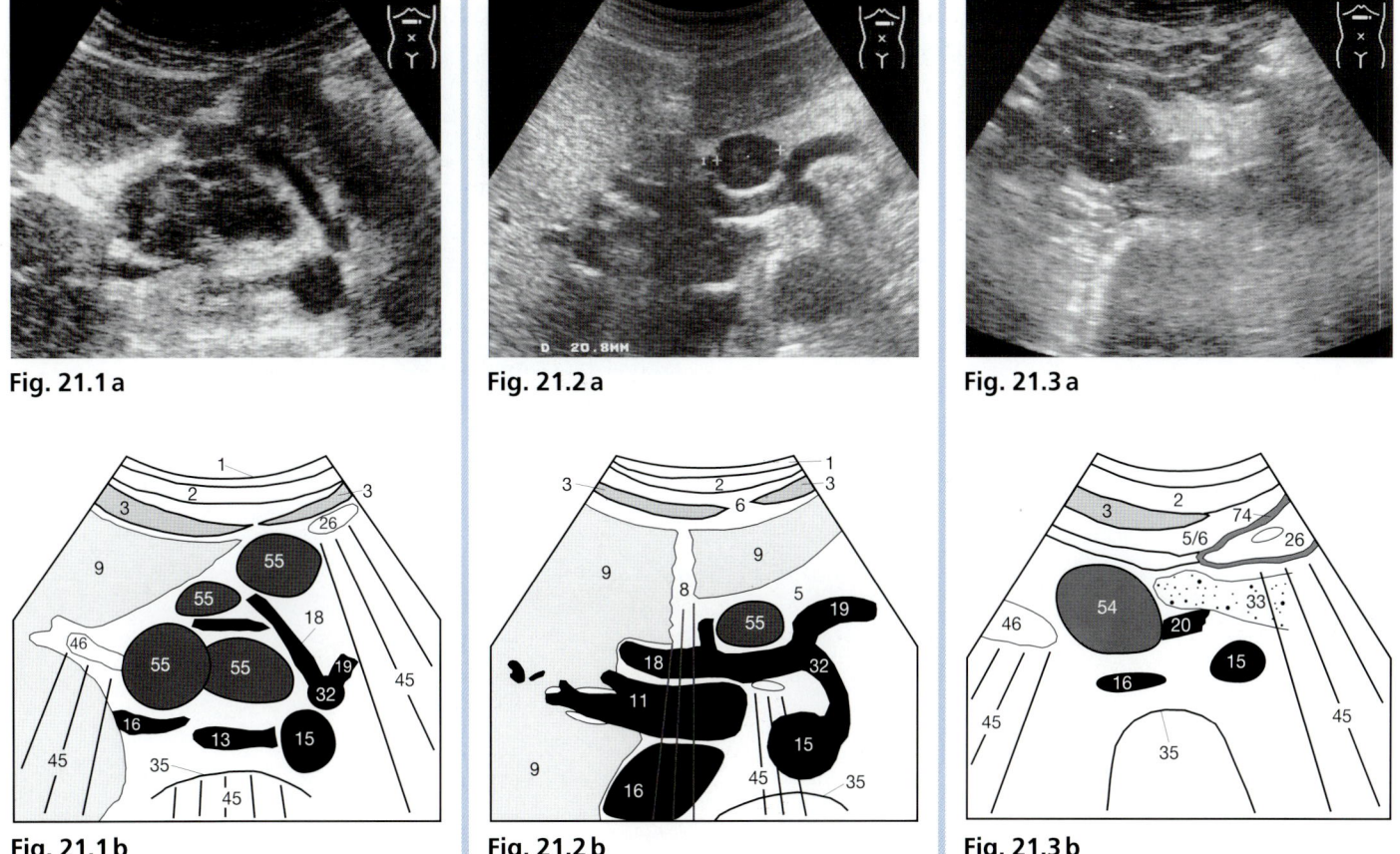

Fig. 21.1 a   Fig. 21.2 a   Fig. 21.3 a

Fig. 21.1 b   Fig. 21.2 b   Fig. 21.3 b

2 Axial Overview — Quiz for Self-Assessment

After this session the standard sagittal and transverse sections are supplemented by oblique sections, clarifying the spatial orientation of individual structures. Answering the subsequent questions correctly is a prerequisite for the next session. The answer to question 4 is found on page 76.

1 Draw the approximate course of the relevant upper abdominal vessels on a piece of paper, naturally just from memory without the help of this workbook. This drawing should include the biliary ducts. Test your knowledge by comparing your drawing with the one shown in **Figure 17.2** and with the key on the unfolded back cover. Repeat this exercise until you succeed without making any mistakes.

2 How does the echogenicity of the pancreas parenchyma increase with advancing age? How is acute pancreatitis recognized? What other imaging modalities are available if sonography fails to delineate the pancreas because of increased bowel gas?

3 Try, without consulting this workbook and entirely from memory, to draw the three standard planes of the upper abdomen. Pay attention to the correct depth dimension of the individual vessels and to accurate annotation! Do not forget the structures of the anterior abdominal wall. Compare your finished sketches with the drawings shown in **Figures 18.1c–18.3c**. Repeat these exercises until you get them right—only then will you have mastered the topographic anatomy of the most important sonographic planes and have laid the foundation for understanding the subsequent oblique sections.

4 On this image, name every vessel and *all* other structures. Which vessel appears distended/congested? What can be the cause? Is this finding pathologic?

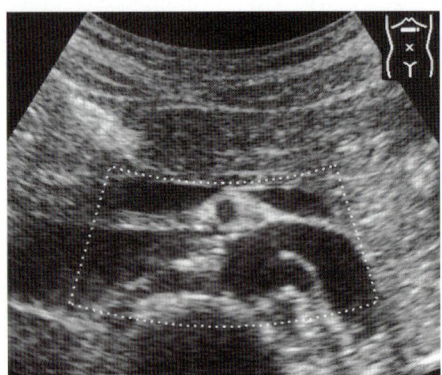

Fig. 22.1

Notes

3 Liver — Porta Hepatis: Normal Findings

This session leaves the transverse plane and moves to a sonographic plane that visualizes the major structures in the lesser omentum. Again, the patient has to be asked to take a deep breath and hold it so that liver and porta hepatis move inferiorly from under the acoustic shadow of the lung and ribs. The transducer is turned from the previous transverse orientation until the sound beam is parallel to the portal vein (roughly parallel to left costal arch) **(Fig. 23.1a)**. Sometimes, the transducer has to be angled craniad **(Fig. 23.1b)** to follow the course of the portal vein **(11)** from the porta hepatis to the confluens of the splenic vein and superior mesenteric vein **(12) (Fig. 23.2)**.

Three hypoechoic layers can be delineated in the minor omentum. The normal position of the portal vein **(11)** is immediately anterior to the obliquely sectioned inferior vena cava **(16)**, with the common bile duct (not visualized in **Fig. 23.2**) and hepatic artery proper **(18)** situated more anterior. Good visualization without intervening duodenal air also allows delineation of the pancreatic head, aorta **(15)**, and SMA **(17)** on the right side of the display (i.e., on the patient's left side).

The major branches of the hepatic artery **(18)** divide at the porta hepatis, with one branch seen in cross-section on the sonographic orientation under discussion here. This cross-section should not be mistaken for preaortic lymphadenopathy **(Fig. 23.2b)**.

The common bile duct can be so narrow that it might be barely visible along the adjacent artery. Its normal diameter should be less than 6 mm. After cholecystectomy it assumes some reservoir function and can dilate up to 9 mm without pathologic significance. A borderline dilated common bile duct (obstructive cholestasis) can no longer be differentiated from adjacent vessels by its luminal diameter but only by its location anterior to the portal vein. Visualizing the duct's entire length is important to exclude intraductal gallstones (see p. 35). By moving the transducer, an attempt should be made to follow all three tubular structures upward to the porta hepatis. Distally, the common bile duct should be followed to the duodenal ampulla at the pancreatic head, the hepatic artery to the celiac axis, and the portal vein to the portosplenic confluence or the splenic vein.

The normal luminal width of the portal vein is less than 13 mm when its main branch is measured perpendicular to its longitudinal axis. Dilatation should only be suspected with measurements exceeding 15 mm. A dilated portal vein alone is an uncertain criterion for the presence of portal hypertension. The highest accuracy is achieved by the definitive demonstration of portocaval collaterals, which are described on the next page.

Normal values:
Portal vein	< 13 mm
Common bile duct	< 6 mm
Common bile duct, S/P cholecystectomy	< 9 mm

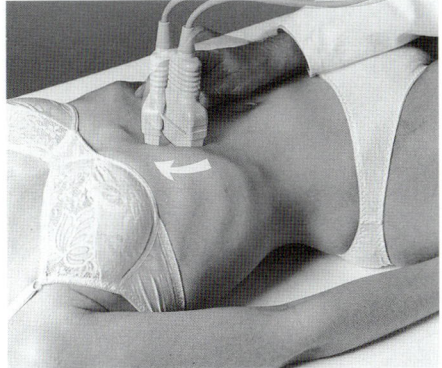
Fig. 23.1a

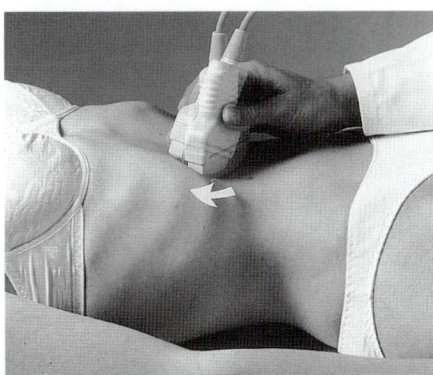
Fig. 23.1b

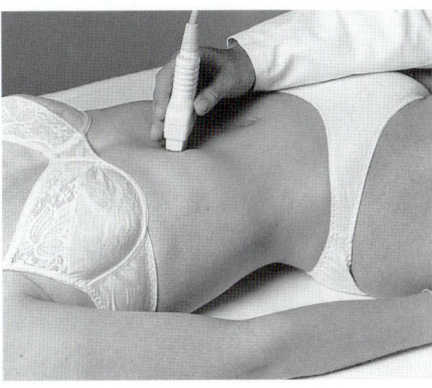
Fig. 23.2a

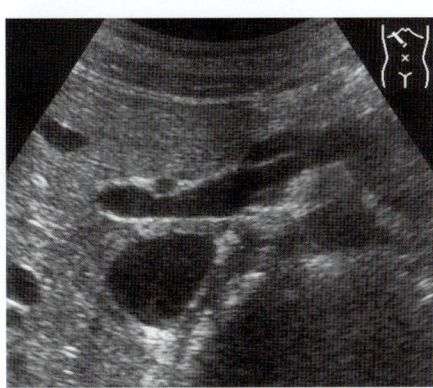
Fig. 23.2b

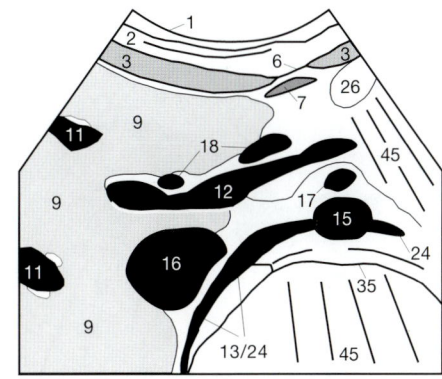
Fig. 23.2c

Liver — Portal Hypertension: Lymph Nodes

The most common cause of increased pressure in the portal vein is impaired drainage secondary to cirrhosis. Direct compression of the portal vein by adjacent tumor is found less frequently. A pancreatic tumor can involve the splenic vein or superior mesenteric vein, without affecting the portal vein. Dilatation of the portal vein (11) to more than 13 mm should be considered suspicious for portal hypertension (Fig. 24.1). The luminal diameter of the portal vein is measured perpendicular to the vessel's longitudinal axis, which is usually obliquely oriented in relation to the sonographic image. The vascular wall is not included in the measurement. It should be kept in mind that splenomegaly of any other cause can lead to an increased luminal diameter of the splenic vein or portal vein, without the presence of portal hypertension.

A dilated portal vein with a diameter of more than 13 mm is by itself no certain criterion for portal hypertension. Additional criteria are splenomegaly (Fig. 48.2), ascites (Fig. 31.1), and portocaval collaterals. With progressing cirrhosis, collateral channels develop to the superior or inferior vena cava. Blood can drain from the portal system via a dilated coronary vein of the stomach and a dilated esophageal venous complex into the (hemi-)azygos vein and from there into the superior vena cava. This can lead to the severe clinical complication of bleeding esophageal varicose veins.

Occasionally, small venous connections between the splenic hilum and left renal vein open up, with resultant portosystemic drainage directly into the inferior vena cava (spontaneous splenorenal shunt). Less frequently, the umbilical vein, which passes through the falciform ligament and ligamentum teres from the porta hepatis to the umbilical vein, recanalizes (Cruveilhier–Baumgarten syndrome). In its advanced stage, this collateral circulation (Fig. 24.2) can produce dilated and markedly tortuous subcutaneous periumbilical veins referred to as caput medusae. In questionable cases, color Doppler sonography can be used to detect a decreased or reversed (hepatofugal) portal blood flow.

Evaluation of the lesser omentum should not only assess the luminal diameter of the portal vein but also exclude enlarged periportal lymph nodes (55) (Fig. 24.3), which frequently accompany viral hepatitis, cholecystitis, or pancreatitis. They are caused by inflammatory changes and should be repeatedly checked for resolution and exclusion of malignant lymphoma.

Checklist Portal Hypertension:

- Demonstration of portocaval collaterals at the porta hepatis
- Diameter of the portal vein at the porta hepatis > 15 mm
- Dilatation of the splenic vein > 1.2 cm
- Splenomegaly
- Demonstration of ascites
- Recanalized umbilical vein (Cruveilhier–Baumgarten syndrome)
- Esophageal varices (by endoscopy)

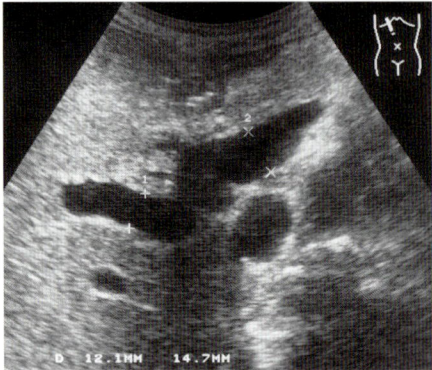

Fig. 24.1 a

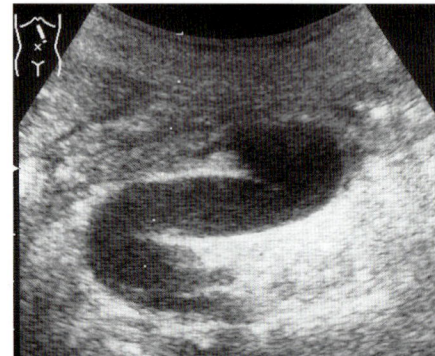

Fig. 24.2 a

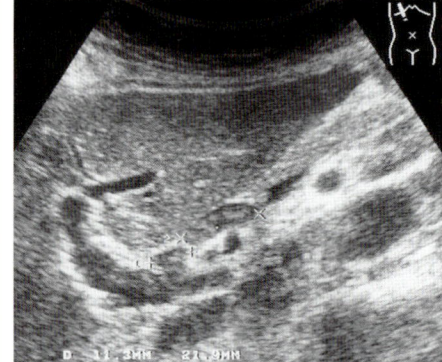

Fig. 24.3 a

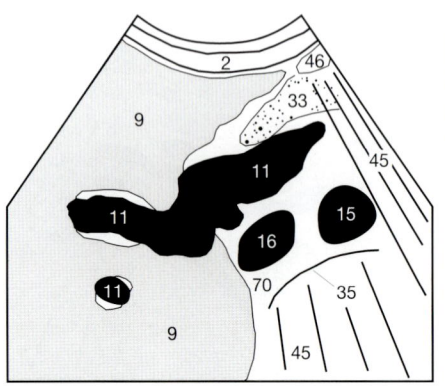

Fig. 24.1 b

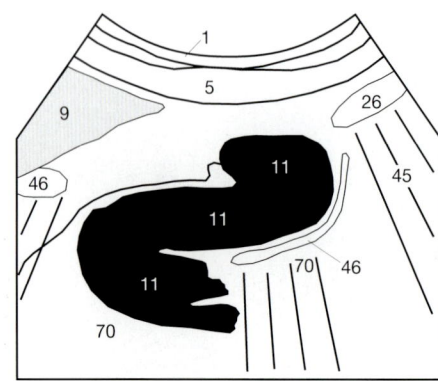

Fig. 24.2 b

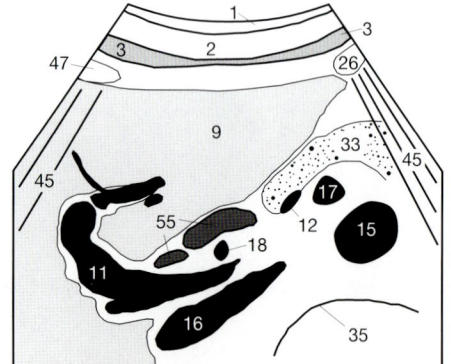

Fig. 24.3 b

3 Liver — Hepatic Vein Confluence and Hepatic Congestion

After the porta hepatis has been evaluated, the liver itself is methodically visualized on transverse images and subcostal oblique images parallel to the right costal arch. What is wrong with the position of the transducer shown in **Fig. 25.1**? The answer can be found in the left lower corner of this page.

The right subcostal oblique image **(Fig. 25.2 a)** is particularly suitable for visualizing the hepatic veins lengthwise **(10)** and their confluence with the obliquely visualized inferior vena cava **(16)**.

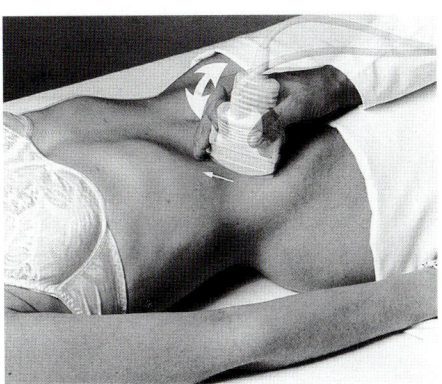

Fig. 25.1

If the inferior vena cava is borderline in diameter and the maneuver to test the caval collapse with forced inspiration is unsuccessful (see p. 15) or inconclusive, the luminal diameter of the hepatic veins is best measured at this level. The maximal diameter of a peripheral hepatic vein should not exceed 6 mm **(Fig. 25.2)**. Measuring the hepatic veins at the confluence with the inferior vena cava has the disadvantage of wide anatomic variations and corresponding false measurements. For instance, the hepatic veins of the patient with no cardiac problems shown in **Fig. 25.2** measure 10 mm directly anterior to the vena cava while the peripheral hepatic veins measure only 3–5 mm. With venous congestion proximal to the right atrium secondary to right-sided heart failure, the hepatic veins are dilated **(Fig. 25.3)** and lack any respiratory changes.

This image section also allows the exclusion of a right pleural effusion, which appears as echo-free fluid between the diaphragm **(13)** and the acoustic shadow of the lung **(47)**. Vascular rarefaction along the periphery of the liver can be a sign of advanced cirrhosis. Hepatic vein thrombosis (Budd–Chiari syndrome) can be diagnosed on the oblique subcostal image with color Doppler sonography, which can determine velocity, profile, and direction of the intravascular blood flow.

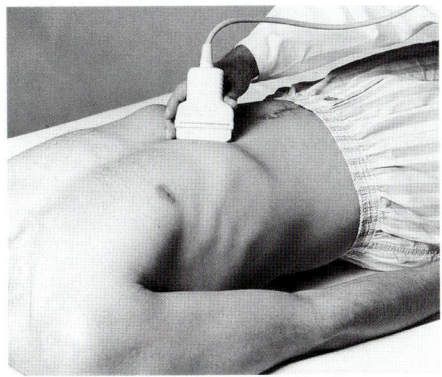

Fig. 25.2 a

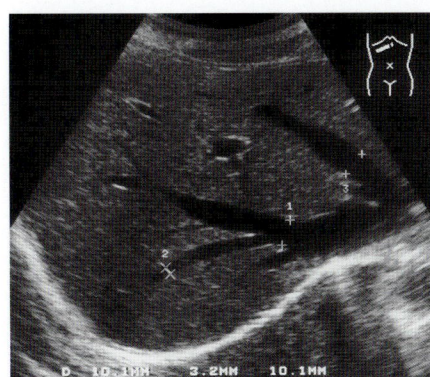

Fig. 25.2 b

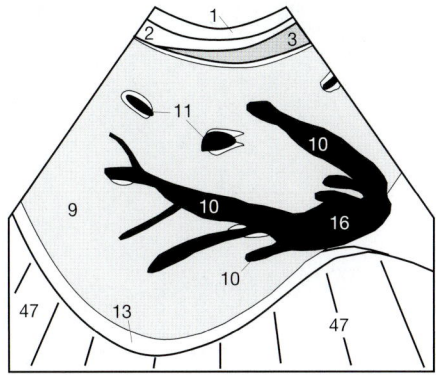

Fig. 25.2 c

Normal values:
Hepatic veins (peripheral):   < 6 mm

Answer to quiz, Fig. 25.1:
The transducer is too far lateroinferior in position. It must be moved towards the costal arch and more medially (see small arrow).

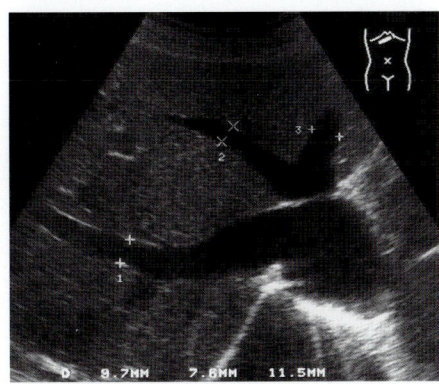

Fig. 25.3 a

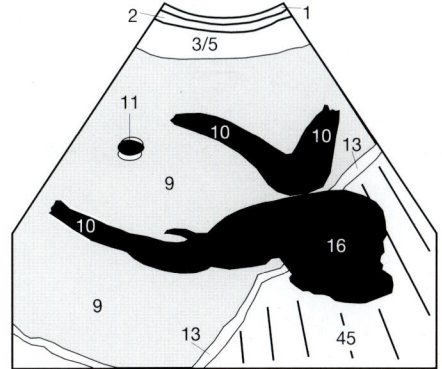

Fig. 25.3 b

3 Liver — Hepatic Size, Gallbladder, Normal Findings

After the liver (9) has been scrutinized on transverse and subcostal image sections, it is further evaluated sagittally, also in deep inspiration (Fig. 26.1a). It is important to keep the patient cooperative by allowing adequate time intervals for normal breathing. The best method seems to be a two-stage evaluation with a slow, continuous sweeping of the transducer. First, the left hepatic lobe is screened to the level of the inferior vena cava, followed by a break for normal breathing while the transducer is moved from the midline to the right MCL. The patient takes another deep breath and the right hepatic lobe is now methodically screened applying the same sweeping motion (Fig. 26.1a) to the transducer.

The size of the liver is assessed by measuring the anteroposterior (sagittal) and the superoinferior diameters in the right MCL (Fig. 26.2a, Fig. 26.3a). To encompass an enlarged liver, the transducer has to be angled superiorly and inferiorly (Fig. 26.1b). Measurements are taken in inspiration. The normal craniocaudal diameter should be less than 13 or 15 cm, depending on the patient's body habitus. It is important to watch for the acute angle formed by the inferior margin of the right hepatic lobe. In hepatic congestion or hepatomegaly, this angle exceeds 45° and becomes blunted. The normal lateral margin of the left hepatic lobe also should form an acute angle measuring less than 30°.

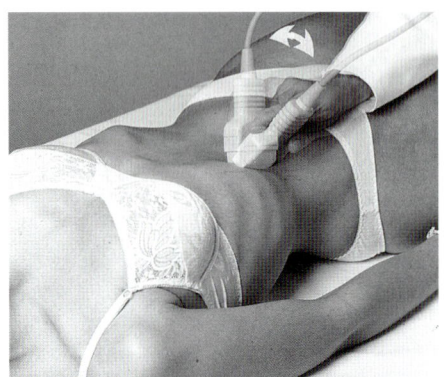

Fig. 26.1 a

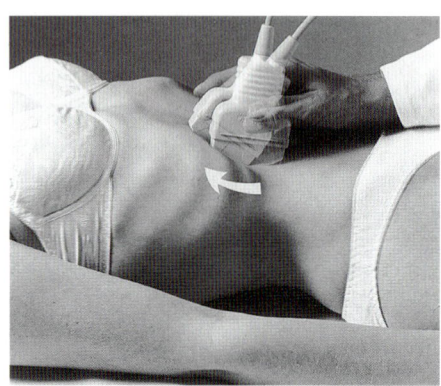

Fig. 26.1 b

The normal gallbladder wall (80), which should only be evaluated when the gallbladder (16) is not contracted (the patient must be NPO), can measure up to 4 mm in thickness (Fig. 26.3). The postprandial gallbladder is generally too contracted to exclude edematous wall thickening, stones, or a tumor with any degree of certainty.

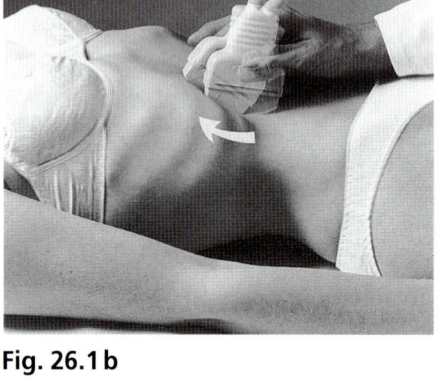

Fig. 26.2 a

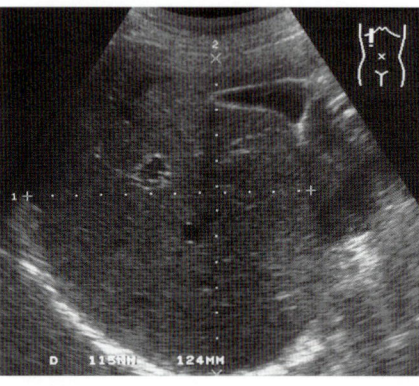

Fig. 26.2 b

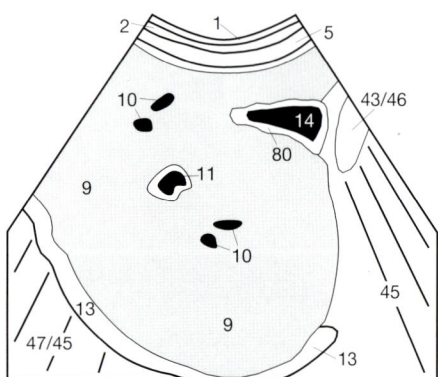

Fig. 26.2 c

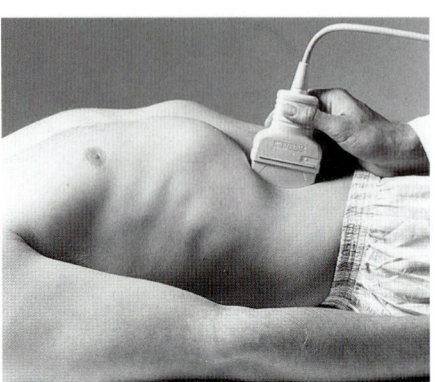

Fig. 26.3 a

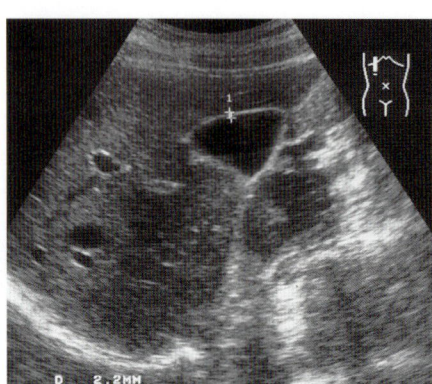

Fig. 26.3 b

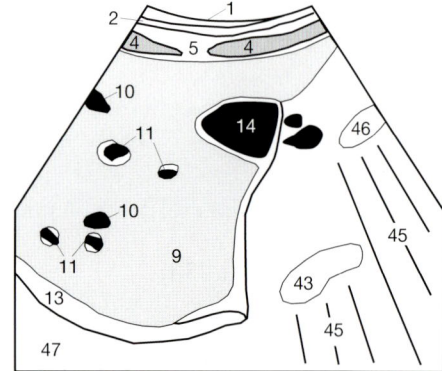

Fig. 26.3 c

3 Liver — Normal Variants, Fatty Liver

In athletic persons, hyperechoic structures (↓) that appear to arise from the concave diaphragmatic surface **(13)** can indent the hepatic dome **(9)** **(Fig. 27.1)**. These structures are only a few millimeters in width and are imprints caused by thickened muscular bundles that run from the central tendon to the costal insertion of the diaphragm. They have no clinical significance and should not be mistaken for pathologic processes. A similar diaphragmatic muscular bundle can also be seen as a mirror artifact along the pulmonary side of the diaphragm **(Fig. 27.2)**.

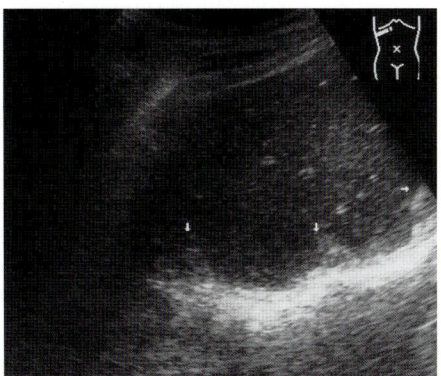

Fig. 27.1 a

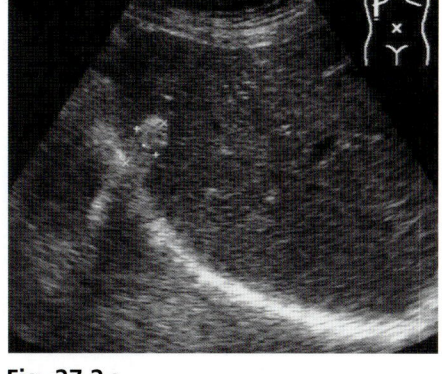

Fig. 27.2 a

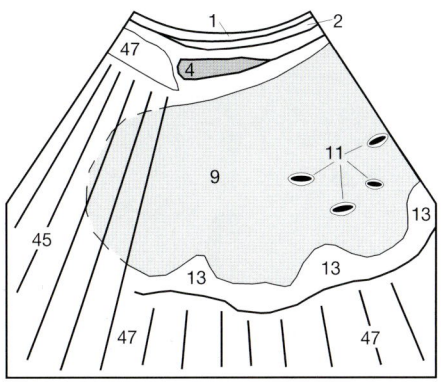

Fig. 27.1 b

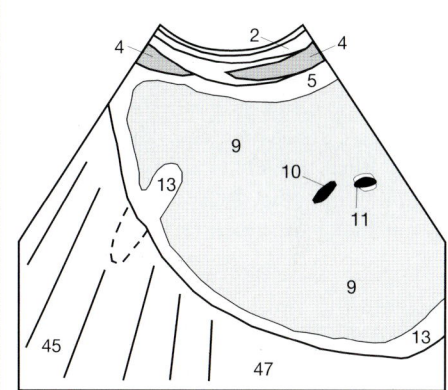

Fig. 27.2 b

A fatty liver or hepatic steatosis produces a diffuse increase in echogenicity of the liver **(Fig. 27.3)**. This increased echogenicity is best appreciated in comparison with the renal echogenicity **(29)**. In normal patients, liver and kidney exhibit about the same echogenicity **(Fig. 37.3)**. The reflection caused by severe hepatic fatty infiltration results in sound attenuation **(Fig. 27.4)** that increases in the liver commensurate with the distance from the transducer. The resultant decreased echogenicity in the more posterior regions of the liver might not be adequate for evaluation. Do you remember why the hepatic parenchyma appears more echogenic behind the gallbladder **(70)**? If not, look it up on page 9.

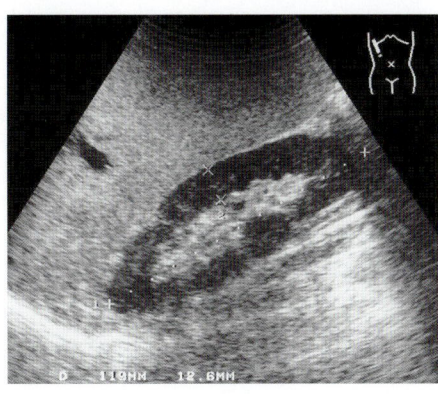

Fig. 27.3 a

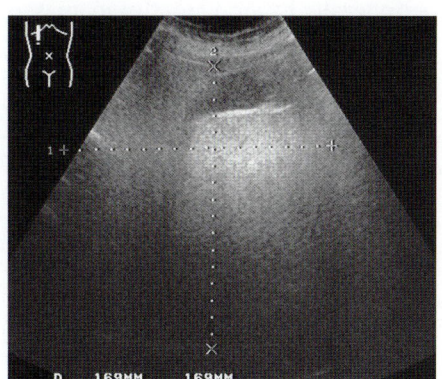

Fig. 27.4 a

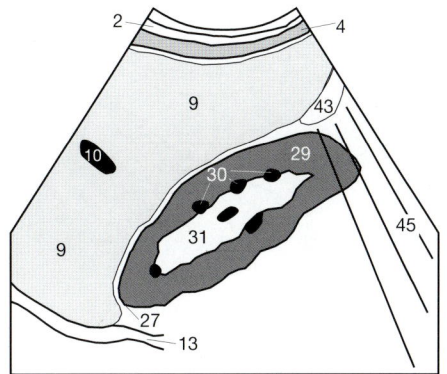

Fig. 27.3 b

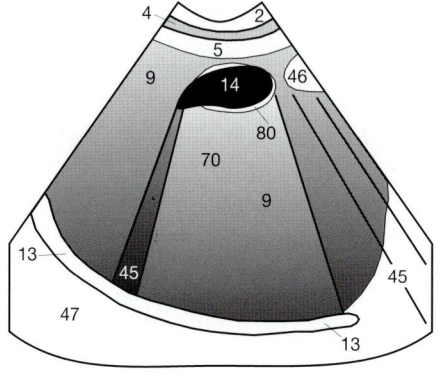

Fig. 27.4 b

3 Liver

Focal Fatty Infiltration

Fatty infiltration is not only diffuse throughout the liver, but may also be confined and regional. These focal fatty changes (63) predominantly occur around the gallbladder fossa or anterior to the portal vein (11). The areas of increased fat content are sharply demarcated and more echogenic than the surrounding hepatic parenchyma (9). They can assume a geographic configuration (Fig. 28.1) and have no space-occupying effect. Adjacent hepatic veins (10) or the branches of the portal veins (11) are not displaced.

The falciform ligament (8), which is composed of connective tissue and surrounded by fat, is seen as a similar echogenic structure that sharply interrupts the adjacent normal hepatic parenchyma (Fig. 28.2). It must be distinguished from focal fatty infiltration.

Diffuse fatty infiltration might not involve the entire liver, resulting in focal fatty sparing (62). These regions of relatively reduced fatty content are primarily found in the immediate vicinity of the portal vein or gallbladder (14) (Fig. 28.4). Again, this finding lacks a space-occupying component. Adjacent vessels are not displaced (Fig. 28.3); peripherally located areas of increased or relatively reduced fatty infiltration show no bulging hepatic border and do not project into the gallbladder, as is sometimes the case with tumors or metastases.

The branches of the portal vein (11) can be distinguished from hepatic veins by their hyperechoic outline. This appearance is caused by the density difference between the portal vein wall, periportal connective tissue, and accompanying biliary duct and hepatic artery. This hyperreflectivity of the portal vein wall (5) becomes accentuated in the vicinity of the porta hepatis (Fig. 28.2) where it should not be mistaken for focal fatty infiltration. Since the hepatic veins (10) traverse the parenchyma without concomitant vessels, they lack a density difference and do not show any wall hyperechogenicity. Only a large hepatic vein perpendicular to the sound beam can exhibit a hyperechogenic wall.

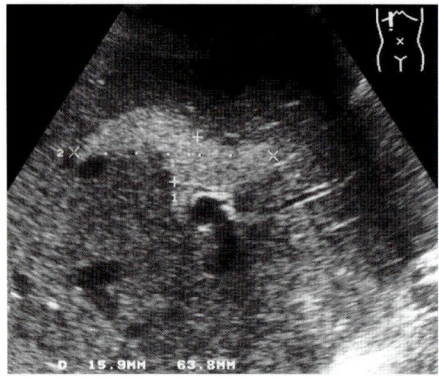

Fig. 28.1 a

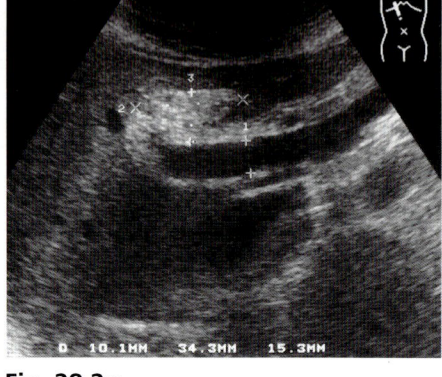

Fig. 28.2 a

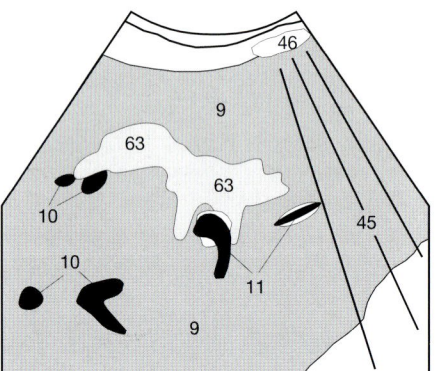

Fig. 28.1 b

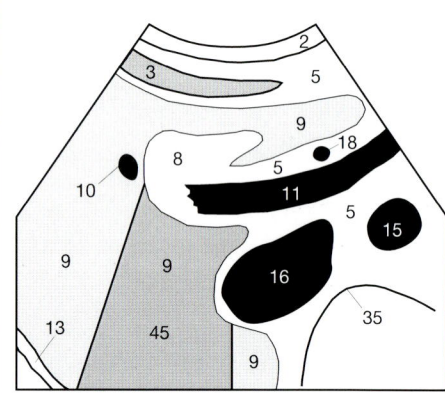

Fig. 28.2 b

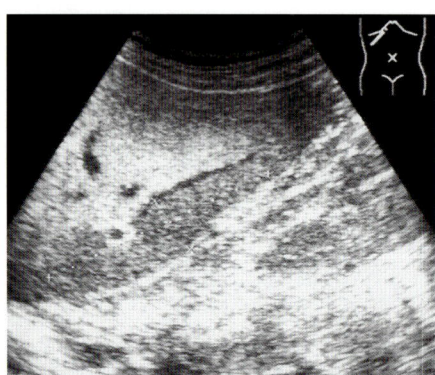

Fig. 28.3 a

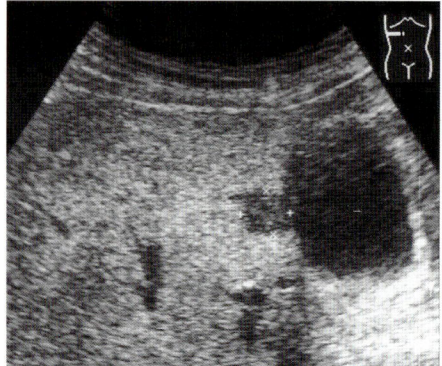

Fig. 28.4 a

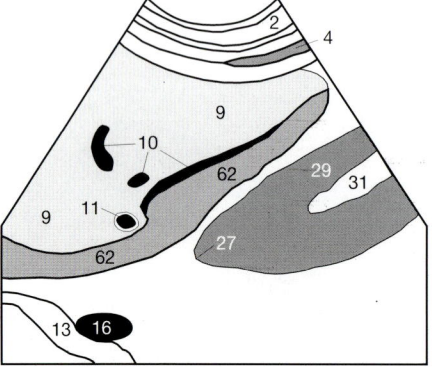

Fig. 28.3 b

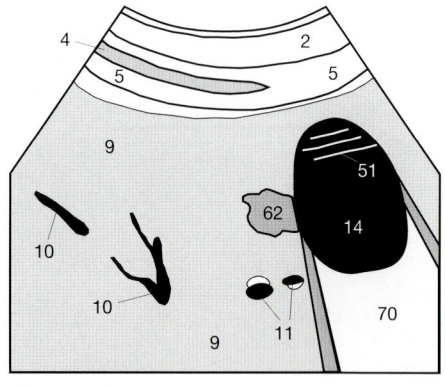

Fig. 28.4 b

3 Liver — Other Focal Changes

Hepatic cysts (64) can be congenital (dysontogenetic) or acquired. In contrast to congenital biliary dilatations (Caroli syndrome), the congenital cysts contain no bile but serous fluid (Fig. 29.1). They are of no clinical consequence unless associated with polycystic kidneys (Fig. 38.3) (risk of renal failure).

The criteria to distinguish a cyst from a lesion of low echogenicity are as follows: echo-free content, spherical shape, smooth outline, distal acoustic enhancement (70), and edge effect (see p. 9). Congenital cysts can exhibit indentations or delicate septa, and parasitic hepatic cysts must then be excluded (Fig. 30.3). Diagnostic difficulties can arise when internal echoes are found secondary to intracystic hemorrhage.

Hepatic hemangiomas (61) are homogeneously echogenic (bright) in comparison to the remaining hepatic tissue (9), have a smooth outline, and lack an echogenic rim. A draining, but not dilated, hepatic vein (10) can be characteristically found in their immediate vicinity (Fig. 29.3). Most hemangiomas are small (Fig. 29.2), but they can reach considerable size and are then generally of rather heterogeneous echogenicity, making it difficult to establish a definitive diagnosis. The lesion (54) shown in (Fig. 29.4) can represent a large hemangioma or malignant tumor, but actually is a focal nodular hyperplasia (FNH), which is not always iso-echoic in relation to the surrounding hepatic parenchyma. Unclear cases can be further evaluated by a dynamic CT with serial images after bolus injection of contrast medium. A hemangioma exhibits a characteristic enhancement and delayed washout. How would you interpret the echo-free areas (68, 69) seen in Figure 29.3b? The answer can be found in the key at the end of this workbook.

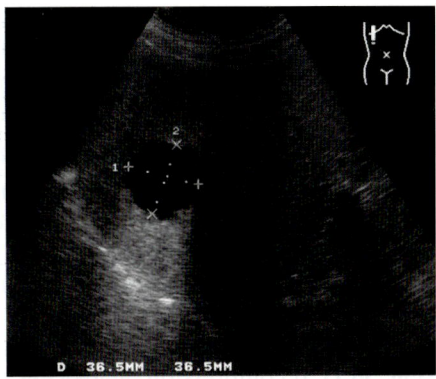

Fig. 29.1 a

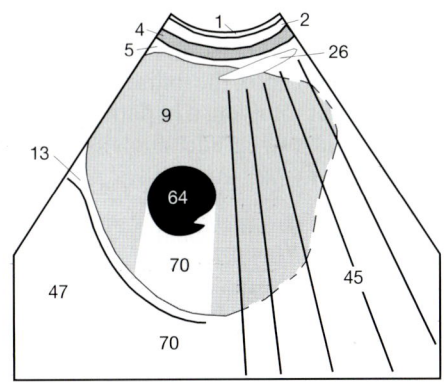

Fig. 29.1 b

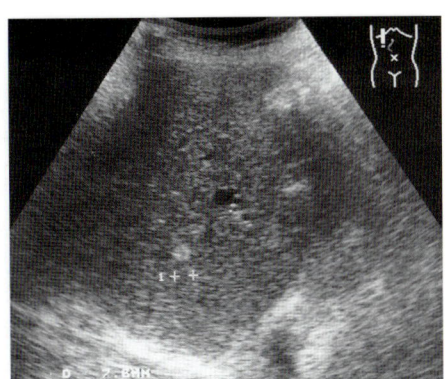

Fig. 29.2 a

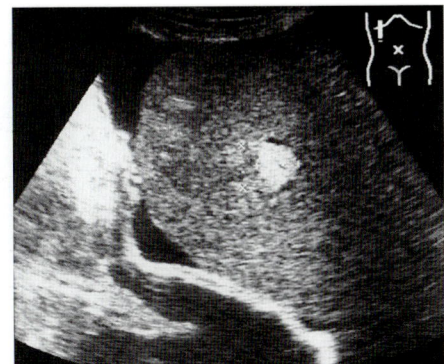

Fig. 29.3 a

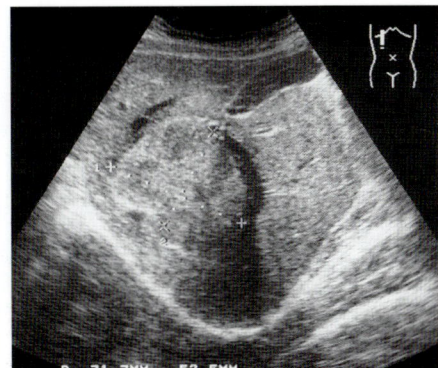

Fig. 29.4 a

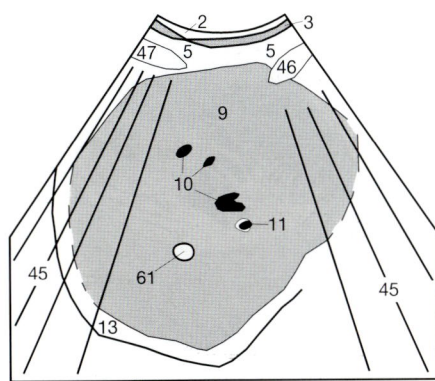

Fig. 29.2 b

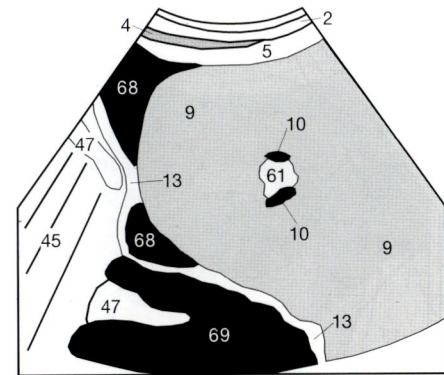

Fig. 29.3 b

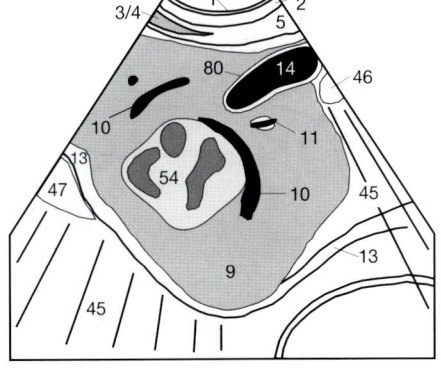

Fig. 29.4 b

Liver — Hepatic Metastases

Secondary neoplastic lesions (metastases) in the liver do not only arise from primary tumors of the intestinal tract, but also from primary tumors in the breast and lung. The sonographic findings are polymorphic. Hepatic metastases (Fig. 32.2) from colorectal carcinomas are often echogenic (56), presumably related to neovascularity secondary to their relatively slow growth. The more rapidly growing metastases from bronchogenic or mammary carcinomas consist almost exclusively of tumor cells and have the tendency to be more hypoechoic. In view of their multifarious presentation, metastases cannot be reliably assigned to any particular primary tumor.

Characteristically, metastases (56) exhibit a hypoechoic halo or rim as seen in Figures 32.1 and 32.2. This hypoechoic zone could represent proliferating tumor or perifocal edema. Central necrosis (57) can frequently be seen as cystic areas caused by liquefaction (Fig. 32.3). Large metastases generally exhibit a space-occupying feature as evidenced by displacement of adjacent vessels. They can compress biliary ducts, possibly leading to regional intrahepatic cholestasis (Fig. 34.2). If located peripherally, they frequently (but not necessarily) expand the hepatic contour that is seen as a localized convexity.

After chemotherapy, various signs of tumor regression can be encountered, such as heterogeneous scars, calcifications, or partial cystic liquefaction, depending on the therapeutic effect. Such regressively altered metastases or small metastatic nodules cannot be easily separated from areas of cirrhotic transformation. It is crucial to follow these findings sonographically to assess their growth potential. Alternatively, a percutaneous needle biopsy under sonographic or CT guidance can be obtained. Multiple metastases that vary in size and echogenicity suggest several episodes of hematogenous spreads.

Do you remember why the hypoechoic bands (45) seen in Figure 32.1 appear in the liver and why the region in between (70) is more echogenic (brighter) than the remaining hepatic parenchyma (9)? Just keep in mind that the gallbladder (14) lies between both findings and the transducer, with the gallbladder wall (80) hit tangentially by the sound beam. If you are still puzzled, you should go back to page 9.

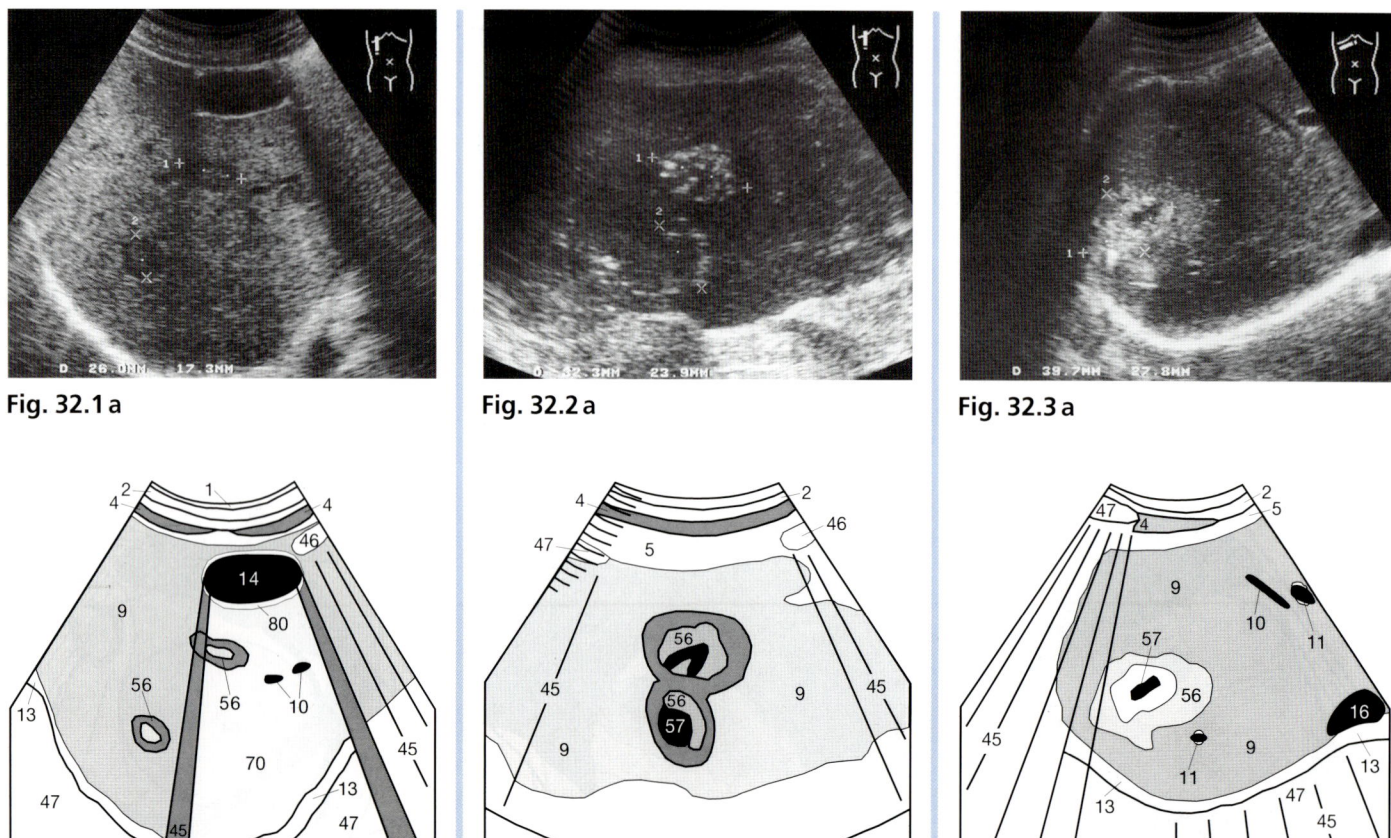

Fig. 32.1 a

Fig. 32.2 a

Fig. 32.3 a

Fig. 32.1 b

Fig. 32.2 b

Fig. 32.3 b

3 Liver — Quiz for Self-Assessment

Before you proceed from the sonographic examination of the liver to the evaluation of the gallbladder, you should try to work through the following questions. The required drawings should be done on a piece of paper. The answers to the questions 6 a–c can be found on page 76, but check the answers only after *all* the questions have been answered so that the suspense does not disappear too early! (You would otherwise inadvertently read the answers to the second and third image questions, that are listed next to each other on page 76.)

1 Try to draw from memory the body marker that shows the section of the porta hepatis. Then make a drawing in the shape of a cone coffee filter and systematically enter from front to back all lines, organs, and vessels that can be expected to appear in this sonographic section. Compare your drawing (but only after completion) with the findings in **Figures 23.2 b and c**. Did you place all major structures in the lesser omentum at the correct depth? If not, repeat this exercise until you succeed without making any mistakes.

2 What is the name of the sonographic section for measuring the luminal diameter of the hepatic vein? Name this section, draw the appropriate body marker, and then proceed as in question 1.

3 What sonographic section is used to measure the liver? What are the maximum diameter values and what are the terms given to them? Can you draw such an image from memory? You already know how to proceed (see above).

4 Write down the three characteristic findings of portal hypertension and the five characteristic findings of cirrhosis. Compare your answers with the material on pages 24 and 31.

5 Name the characteristic sites of focally decreased and focally increased fatty infiltration of the liver. How can they be differentiated from malignant hepatic processes?

6 Review the following three sonographic images. Write down the imaging plane and list your differential diagnosis of the findings. Include *every* abnormality since several pathologic processes are present.

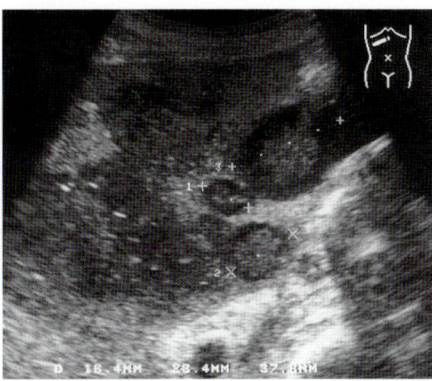

Fig. 33.1

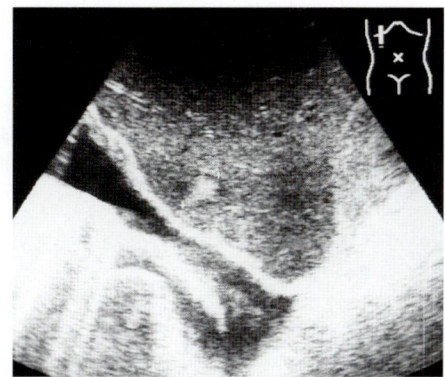

Fig. 33.2

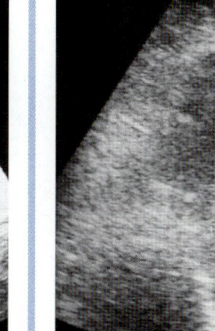

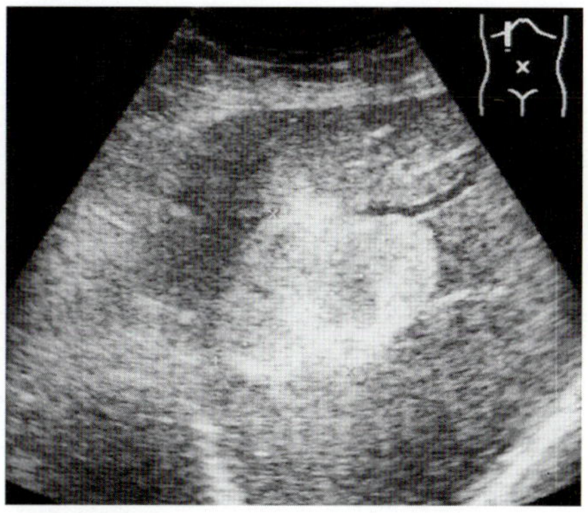

Fig. 33.3

4 Gallbladder and Biliary Ducts — Cholestasis

The bile duct (66), comprising the common hepatic duct above the cystic duct insertion and the common bile duct below it, normally measures up to 6 mm at the level of the minor omentum, but luminal diameters between 7 and 9 mm are still within the range of normal (Fig. 34.1), particularly after cholecystectomy. A dilated duct (exceeding 9 mm in diameter) invariably becomes visible anterolaterally to the portal vein (11) (compare p. 23). Even when the distal segment of the common bile duct is obscured by duodenal air (compare Fig. 17.3), a proximal intrahepatic obstruction (e.g., hepatic metastasis) can be sonographically distinguished from a distal obstruction (e.g., stone lodged at the papilla, lymphadenopathy in the lesser omentum, or carcinoma of the pancreas). The proximal obstruction distends neither gallbladder (14) nor common bile duct.

The small intrahepatic biliary ducts are parallel to the portal vein branches (11) and are normally invisible. They become visible along the portal veins when biliary obstruction has dilated the ducts, resulting in the double-barreled shot-gun sign (Fig. 35.3). Sonography is successful in up to 90% of cases in distinguishing between obstructive (ductal dilatation) and hepatocellular (no ductal dilatation) jaundice. Characteristically, a severe biliary obstruction (Fig. 34.2) produces a tortuous dilatation of the intrahepatic biliary ducts (66) that can assume the appearance of a towering antler. Cholestasis can increase the viscosity of the bile that can lead to the precipitation of cholesterol or calcium crystals (Fig. 34.3). This so-called "sludge" (67) can also be seen after prolonged fasting without biliary obstruction. Before diagnosing sludge, a thickness artifact (p. 10) should be excluded by obtaining additional sections and by turning and shaking the patient. The ERCP can drain a biliary obstruction by inserting a biliary stent (59). Alternatively, biliary drainage can be achieved with a percutaneous transhepatic catheter.

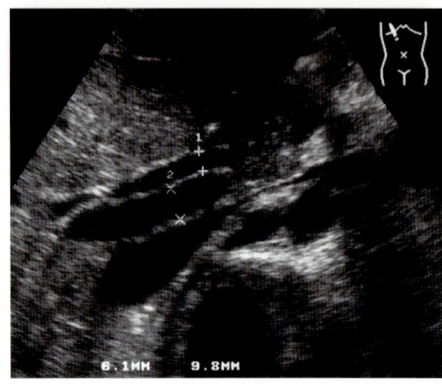

Fig. 34.1 a

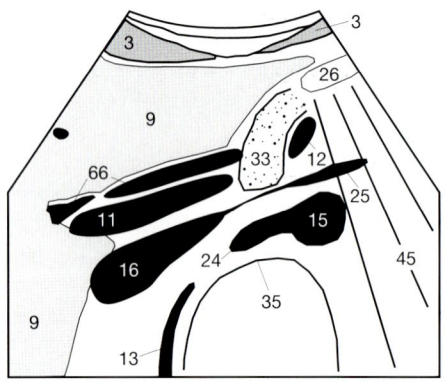

Fig. 34.1 b

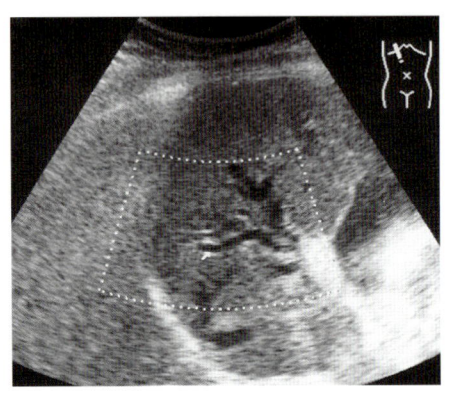

Fig. 34.2 a

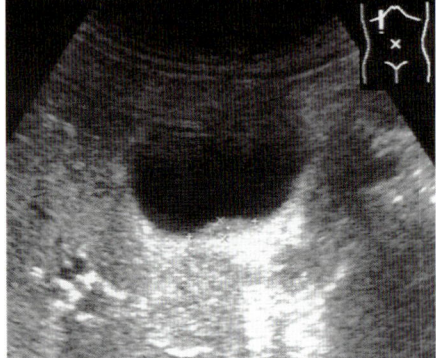

Fig. 34.3 a

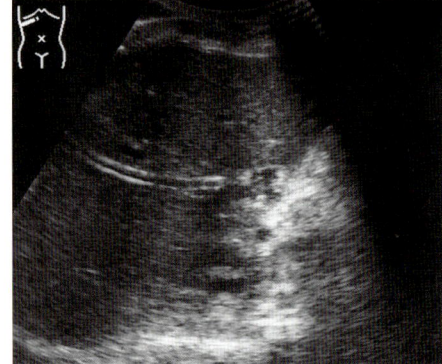

Fig. 34.4 a

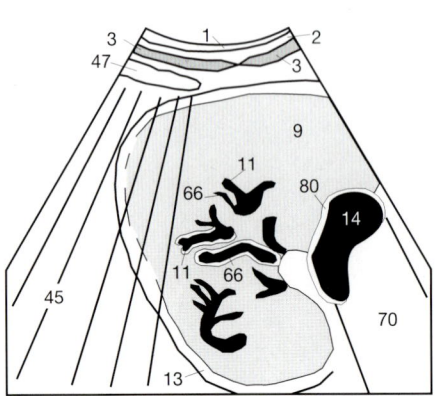

Fig. 34.2 b

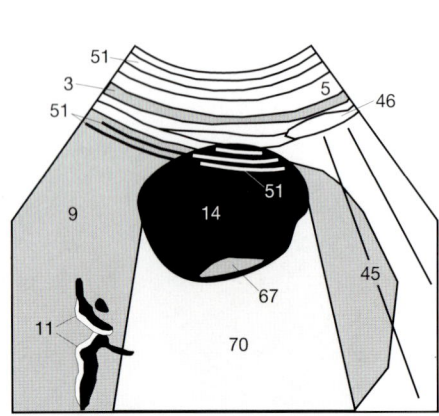

Fig. 34.3 b

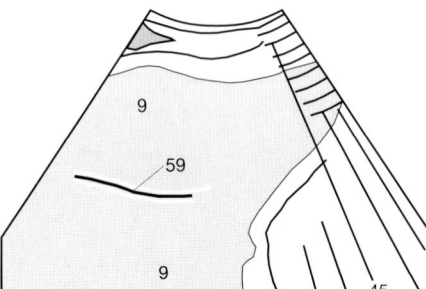

Fig. 34.4 b

4 Gallbladder and Biliary Ducts — Gallstones and Polyps

Stones are formed in the gallbladder (gallstones) because of an altered composition of the excreted bile. Depending on their composition, gallstones **(49)** can transmit sound almost completely **(Fig. 35.3)**, float within the gallbladder (cholesterol stones) or, if high in calcium content, reflect sound to the degree that only the surface is visualized **(Fig. 35.1)**. A stone is established if an echogenic structure can be dislodged from the gallbladder wall **(80)** by moving and turning the patient, in contradistinction to a polyp **(65) (Fig. 35.2)**.

Some stones remain fixed at the gallbladder wall because of inflammatory processes, or become lodged in the infundibulum, rendering the differentiation between stones and polyps difficult. Acoustic shadowing **(45)** distal to such a lesion **(Figs. 35.1, 35.3)** indicates a stone. An edge effect of the gallbladder wall **(45) (Fig. 35.2)** must be carefully distinguished from stone-induced acoustic shadowing **(compare Fig. 9.4)** to avoid any misinterpretation. The polyp shown in this case **(Fig. 35.2)** should be followed for signs of growth to exclude any malignant process.

Intrahepatic cholestasis **(Fig. 34.2)** is not always a manifestation of malignancy and can be caused by obstructing stones **(49)** in the intrahepatic ducts **(66) (Fig. 35.3)**. The prevalence of cholelithiasis is about 15%, whereby older women are affected more often. Since 80% of the patients with gallstones are asymptomatic, detected gallstones are only consequential in context with their complications (cholecystitis, cholangitis, colics, biliary obstruction). If removal is indicated, this can be achieved by percutaneous or open cholecystectomy or, alternatively, by ESWL (extracorporeal shock wave lithotripsy) or ERCP. Furthermore, the composition of the bile can be altered by medication and some stones regress following nutritional changes.

Note the thin, single-layered, echogenic wall **(80)** of both gallbladders **(14)** shown in **Figures 35.1 and 35.2**. There is no inflammatory thickening of the gallbladder wall. Compare this finding to the one on the images on the next page.

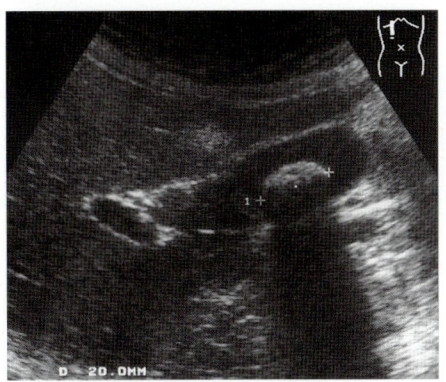

Fig. 35.1 a

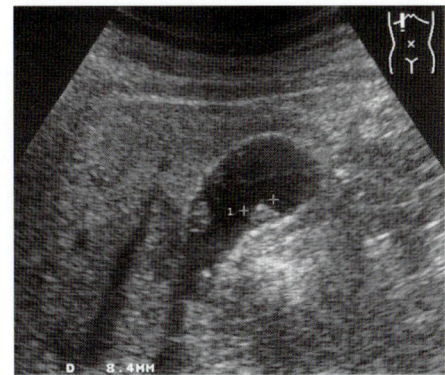

Fig. 35.2 a

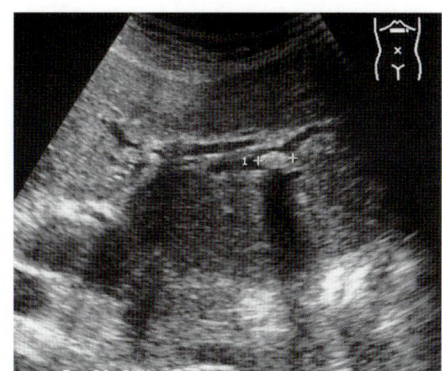

Fig. 35.3 a

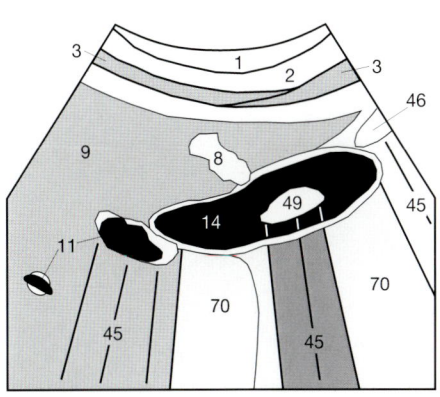

Fig. 35.1 b

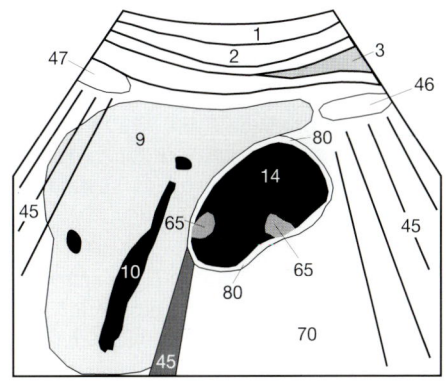

Fig. 35.2 b

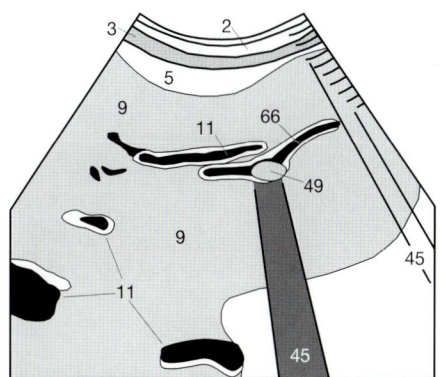

Fig. 35.3 b

4 Gallbladder and Biliary Ducts — Cholecystitis and Quiz for Self-Assessment

Cholecystitis is invariably caused by stones (49). Early cholecystitis only causes the gallbladder (14) to be tender, but inflammatory edema of the gallbladder wall (80) soon develops and the wall becomes thickened and multilayered (Fig. 36.1).

The preprandial gallbladder wall normally measures less than 4 mm. Thickening of the gallbladder wall does not have to be a sign of inflammation since it can be found in many conditions, including ascites (68) (Fig. 36.2), hypoalbuminemia, or right-sided cardiac insufficiency.

An additional finding indicative of an acute inflammation is pericholecystic accumulation of fluid (68), which in some cases can be confined to Morrison's pouch between the inferior hepatic border and right kidney. Finally, the gallbladder can become indistinct in outline where it abuts the hepatic parenchyma (9). An increased diameter of the gallbladder of more than 4 cm is a sign of hydrops, but even more characteristic for hydrops is the associated altered configuration from a pear-shaped to a more biconvex and spherical structure.

Recognizing air within the lumen of the gallbladder or in its wall (mural emphysema) is crucial since an infection with gas-forming organisms implies a poor prognosis and is associated with a high risk of perforation. Chronic cholecystitis can lead to a contracted gallbladder or a porcelain gallbladder with mural calcifications. Both conditions cannot easily be differentiated by sonography and have to be evaluated together with the clinical findings.

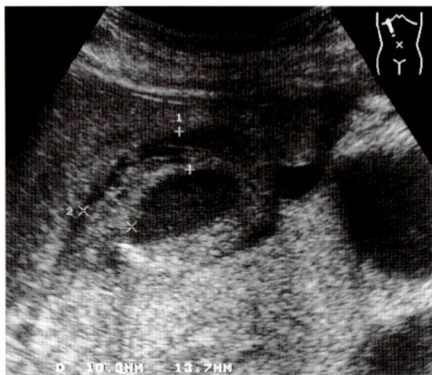

Fig. 36.1 a

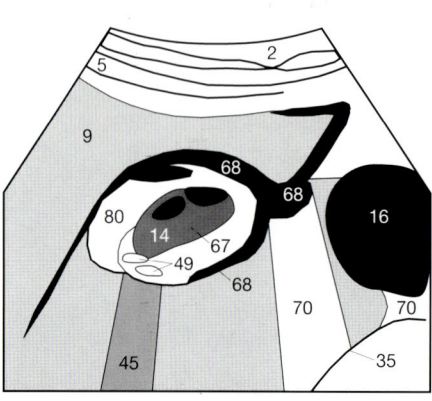

Fig. 36.1 b

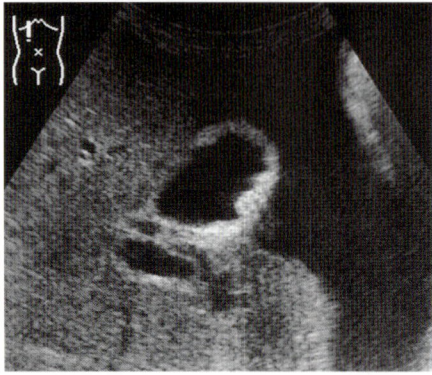

Fig. 36.2 a

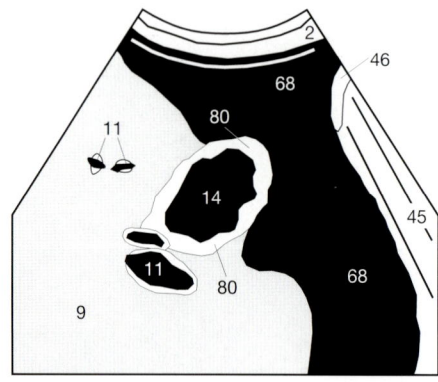

Fig. 36.2 b

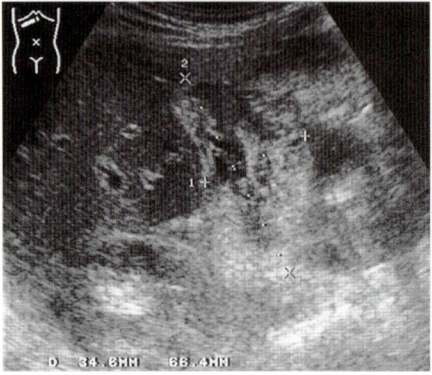

Fig. 36.3

Quiz for self-assessment:

1. What is the maximum diameter of the common bile duct? What diameter in mm arouses suspicion of a biliary obstruction?

2. Write down several diagnoses found in the sonographic image on the left, after careful review. Compare your result with the answer on page 76.

5 Kidneys and Adrenal Glands — Normal Findings

The kidneys are generally best shown in the lateral decubitus position. The longitudinal section of the kidney is visualized by placing the transducer on the extended intercostal line of the flank. With deep inspiration, the kidney moves inferiorly away from the obscuring costal acoustic shadows and appears in its longitudinal dimension (Fig. 37.1 a) for evaluation. As is essential for a complete evaluation of any organ, the kidney must also be delineated in a second plane, as demonstrated in Figure 37.1 b for the evaluation of the transverse plane of the left kidney (right lateral decubitus position).

Normal renal parenchyma (29) is slightly decreased or equal in echogenicity relative to the splenic or hepatic parenchyma (9). The width of the parenchyma should measure at least 1.3 cm (the measurements in Fig. 37.2 are 1.5 cm and 2.4 cm, respectively). The ratio between parenchymal width and pelvic width (= PP-index) decreases with age (compare normal values below). In the typical longitudinal section (Fig. 37.2), the hypoechoic medullary pyramids (30) are seen like a string of pearls between the parenchymal cortex and the centrally situated echogenic collecting system (renal pelvis, 31). They should not be mistaken for tumors or cysts. An enlarged adrenal gland should be searched for within the perirenal fat above the upper pole of the kidney (27), where it can appear as a hypoechoic mass within the echogenic perirenal fat. The renal hilum, together with the renal vein (25), is generally well seen on the transverse section (Fig. 37.3). Because of their thin diameter, the ureter and renal artery are often identified only with great difficulty. Why is the position of the transducer depicted in Figure 37.3 a not completely compatible with the images shown in Figures 37.3 b and c?

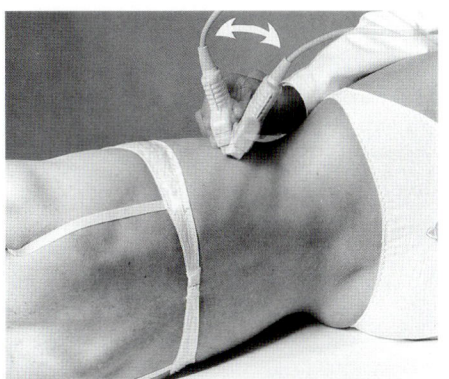

Fig. 37.1 a

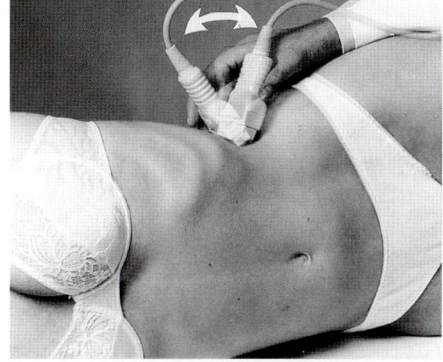

Fig. 37.1 b

Normal renal values:

Renal length:	10–12 cm
Renal width:	4– 6 cm
Respiratory mobility:	3– 7 cm
Parenchymal width:	1.3–2.5 cm
PP-index (depending on age):	
< 30 years:	1.6:1
< 60 years:	1.2–1.6:1
> 60 years	1.1:1

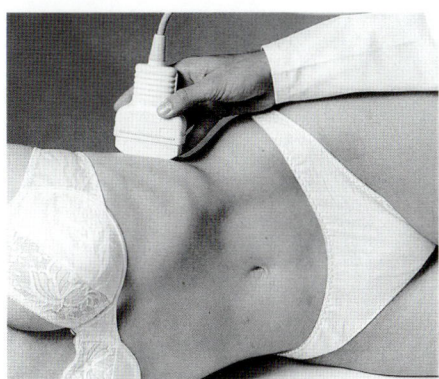

Fig. 37.2 a

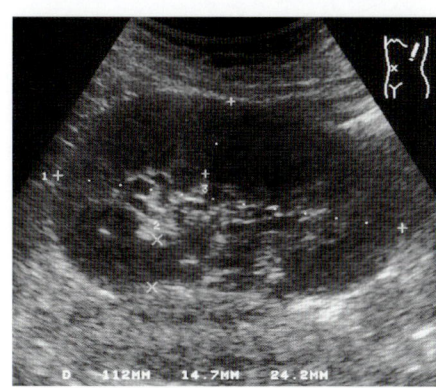

Fig. 37.2 b

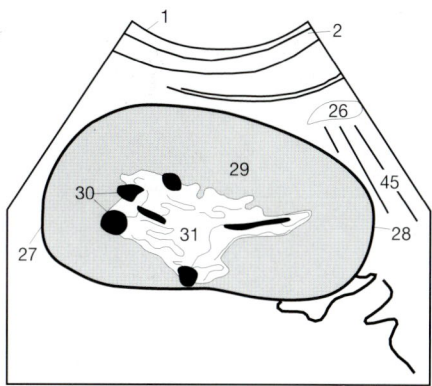

Fig. 37.2 c

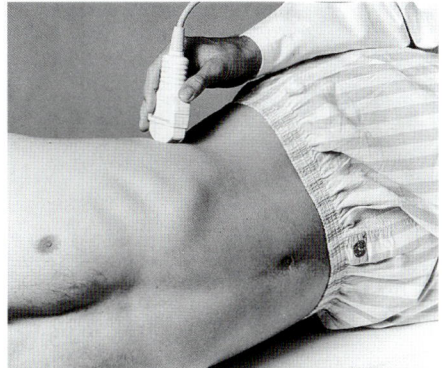

Fig. 37.3 a

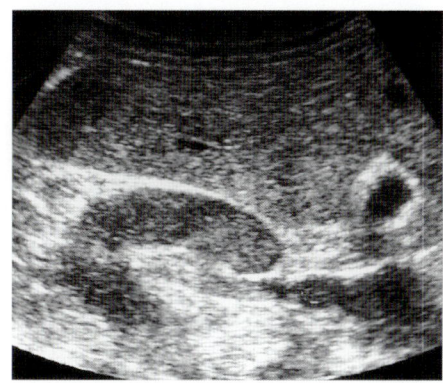

Fig. 37.3 b

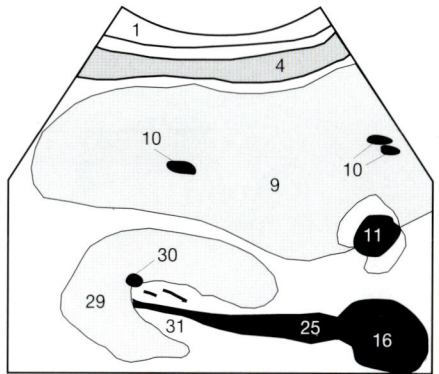

Fig. 37.3 c

5 Kidneys — Normal Variants and Cysts

The normal configuration of the kidney (Fig. 37.2) can show several findings that can be traced to its embryologic development. Hyperplastic columns of Bertin can protrude from the parenchyma (29) into the renal pelvis (31) and do not differ in echogenicity from the remaining renal parenchyma. An equally iso-echogenic parenchymal bridge can completely divide the collecting system. A partial or complete parenchymal gap at the same location indicates a renal duplication (Fig. 38.1) with separate ureters and blood supply for each moiety. The prevertebral parenchymal bridge of horseshoe kidneys might even be mistaken at first sight for preaortic lymphadenopathy or a thrombosed aortic aneurysm. A lobulated renal contour can be seen in children and young adults as manifestation of persistent fetal lobulation, characterized by an otherwise smooth renal surface that is indented between the individual medullary pyramids. These changes have to be differentiated from renal infarcts (Fig. 42.3) that can be found in old patients with atherosclerotic stenosis of the renal artery.

Localized parenchymal thickening along the lateral border of the left kidney, usually just below the inferior pole of the spleen, is found in about 10% of patients. This is an anatomic variant, generally referred to as "dromedary hump," and its differentiation from a true renal tumor might occasionally be difficult.

Renal cysts (64) are echo-free and produce, as shown in Figure 38.2, distal acoustic enhancement (70). Additional criteria for the diagnosis of a cyst are the same as for the diagnosis of hepatic cysts (see p. 29). Cysts can be separated into peripheral cysts along the renal surface, parenchymal cysts, or peripelvic cysts, with the latter to be differentiated from an obstructed and dilated renal pelvis (Fig. 41.2). The evaluation of a cyst should include measuring its diameter as well as stating its approximate location (upper, middle, or lower third of the kidney).

Finding a few renal cysts is clinically inconsequential, though re-evaluation at regular intervals is advisable. In contrast, the adult form of polycystic renal disease (Fig. 38.3) presents with innumerable cysts (64) that progressively increase in size. Since the cysts can reach a considerable size, the patients can complain of fullness and pressure in the upper abdomen. Furthermore, polycystic renal disease leads to renal atrophy by displacing and thinning the renal parenchyma, resulting in renal insufficiency in early adulthood and eventually requiring dialysis or a renal transplant. Other causes of renal atrophy will be discussed on the next page.

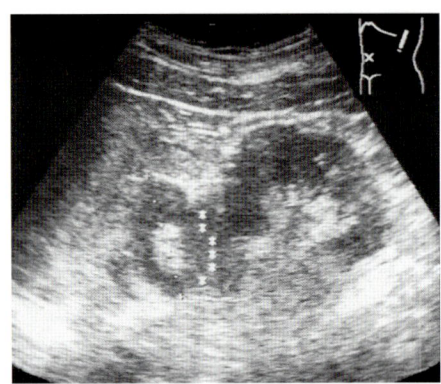

Fig. 38.1 a

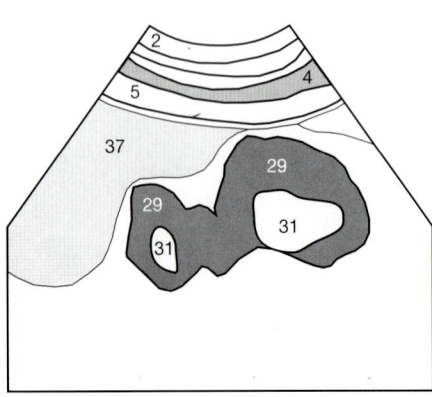

Fig. 38.1 b

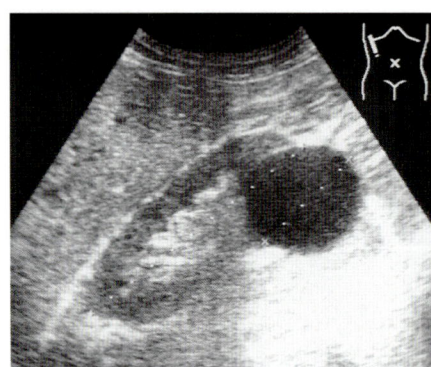

Fig. 38.2 a

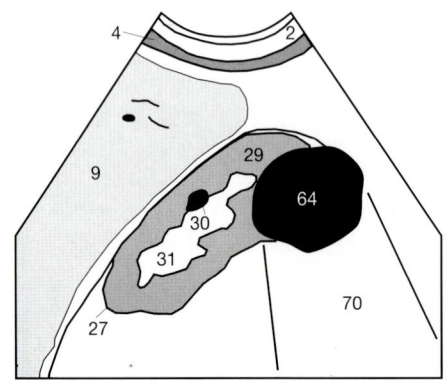

Fig. 38.2 b

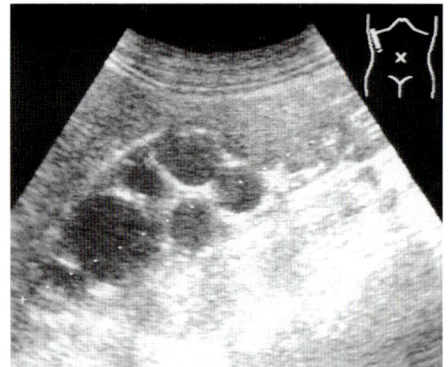

Fig. 38.3 a

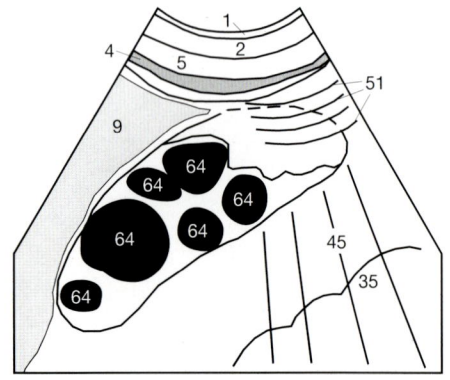

Fig. 38.3 b

5 Kidneys — Atrophy and Inflammation

The kidney reacts to the various inflammatory conditions with similar sonographic changes. It can be entirely normal in early pyelonephritis or glomerulonephritis. Later, edema causes an enlargement and interstitial infiltration an increased parenchymal echogenicity with accentuated demarcation of the parenchyma **(29)** relative to the hypoechoic pyramids **(30)** **(Fig. 39.3)**. This is referred to as "punched-out medullary pyramids." In comparison with the adjacent hepatic or splenic parenchyma **(9)**, the renal parenchyma appears more echogenic **(Fig. 39.3)** than the parenchyma of the normal kidney **(Fig. 38.2)**. Interstitial nephritis can be caused by chronic glomerulonephritis, diabetic nephropathy, urate nephropathy (hyperuricemia as manifestation of gout or increased nucleic acid turnover), amyloidosis or autoimmune disease, but the etiology cannot be deduced from the increased parenchymal echogenicity.

Another sign indicating an inflammation is the indistinct interface between parenchyma and collecting system.

In addition to causing peripheral infarcts **(Fig. 42.3)**, renal artery stenosis can induce a generalized decrease in renal size **(Fig. 39.1)**, which, however, can also be a manifestation of recurrent or chronic inflammation. The marked thinning of the parenchyma **(29)** found in end-stage chronic nephritis leads to renal atrophy **(Fig. 39.2)**, which is frequently accompanied by degenerative calcifications **(53)** or concrements **(49)** with their corresponding acoustic shadows **(45)**. The atrophic kidney can be so small that it eludes sonographic detection. The associated loss of excretory function can be made up by compensatory hypertrophy of the contralateral kidney. In a unilaterally small kidney, the PP index (see p. 37) should be determined. If this index is normal, a developmentally hypoplastic kidney might be present.

While sonography does not contribute to the differential diagnosis of inflammatory renal disease, it is of value in monitoring any renal inflammation during therapy, in excluding any complications (e.g., acute obstruction) and in guiding any percutaneous needle biopsy.

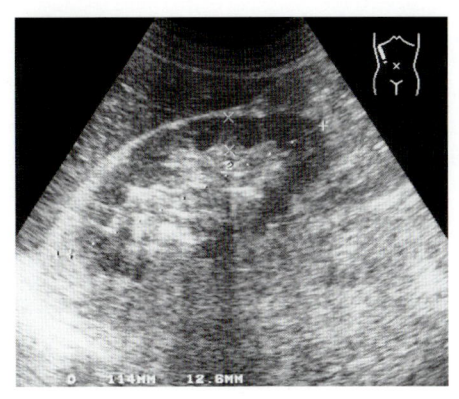

Fig. 39.1 a

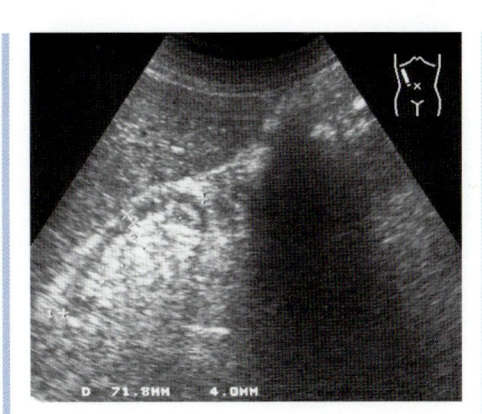

Fig. 39.2 a

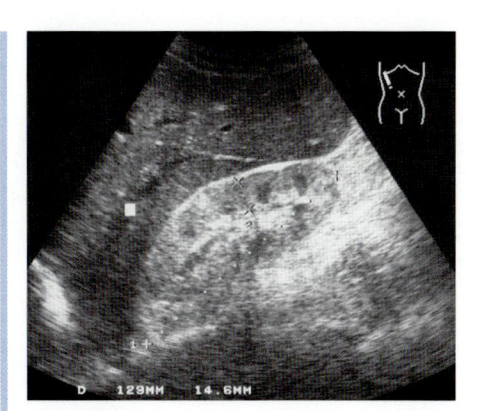

Fig. 39.3 a

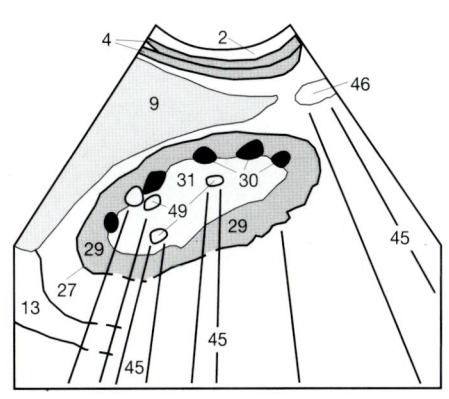

Fig. 39.1 b

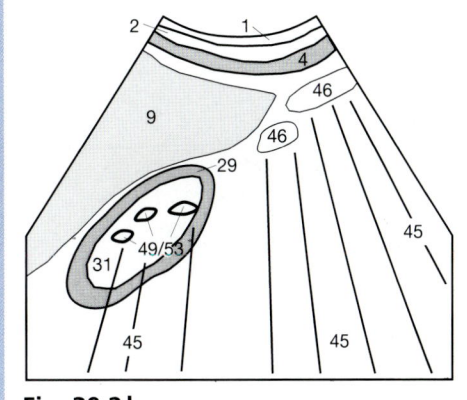

Fig. 39.2 b

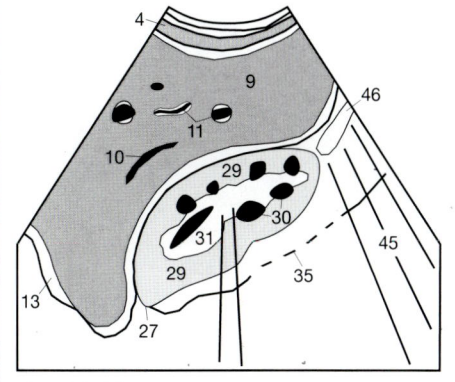

Fig. 39.3 b

5 Kidneys — Urinary Obstruction

The collecting system is seen as a central complex of strong echoes that are only traversed by small thin vascular structures **(Fig. 37.2)**. With increased diuresis after fluid intake, the renal pelvis **(31)** can distend and be visualized as a more echo-free structure **(87)** **(Fig. 40.1)**. The same finding can represent the developmental variant of an extrarenal pelvis. In both conditions, the dilation does not involve the calices and infundibula.

It can be difficult to separate this finding from a first degree (mild) obstructive dilatation **(Fig. 40.2)**, which also causes a dilated renal pelvis but without infundibular extension and detectable parenchymal thinning. A second degree (moderate) obstructive dilatation causes increasing fullness of the infundibula and calices as well as the onset of parenchymal thinning **(Fig. 40.3)**. The bright central echo complex **(31)** becomes rarefied and eventually disappears. The third degree (severe) obstructive dilatation is characterized by severe pressure atrophy of the parenchyma (no case illustrated).

Sonography cannot reveal all the causes of an obstructive uropathy. Since the midureter is obscured by overlying air in the majority of cases, a ureteral stone is generally not visualized unless it is lodged at the ureteropelvic junction or in the prevesical ureter. Less frequent causes of ureteral obstruction are a tumor of the bladder or uterus and aggregated lymph nodes as well as retroperitoneal fibrosis after radiation, or idiopathic as a manifestation of Ormond disease. A latent obstruction can develop during pregnancy, caused by ureteral atony, and during infection. Furthermore, an overdistended bladder as manifestation of a neurogenic bladder or secondary to prostatic hypertrophy can cause ureteral obstruction, and the sonographic evaluation must include the bladder and a search for an enlarged prostate gland in men **(compare Figs. 56.1, 56.2)**. For assessing the postvoid residual see page 54.

The obstruction causing the dilatation of the collecting system can be relieved by cystoscopically placed ureteral stents **(compare Figs. 45.3, 45.4)** or by sonographically guided percutaneous nephrostomy.

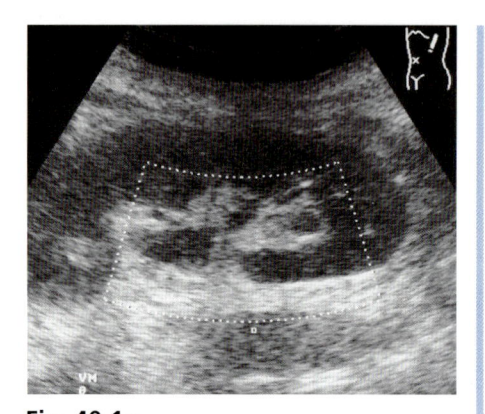

Fig. 40.1 a

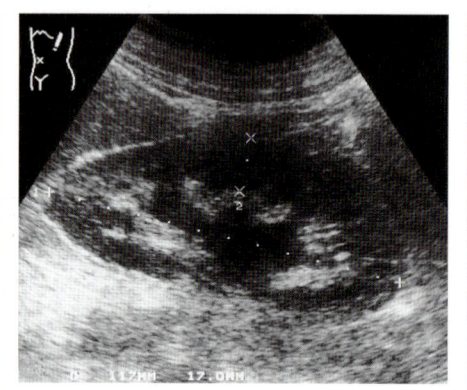

Fig. 40.2 a

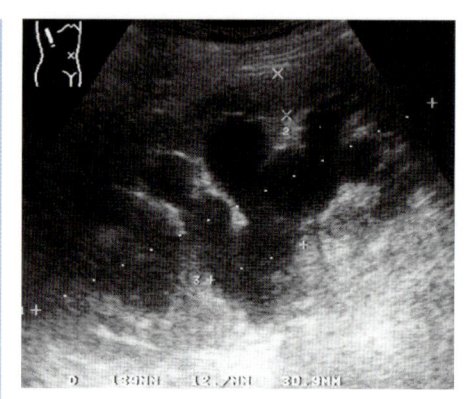

Fig. 40.3 a

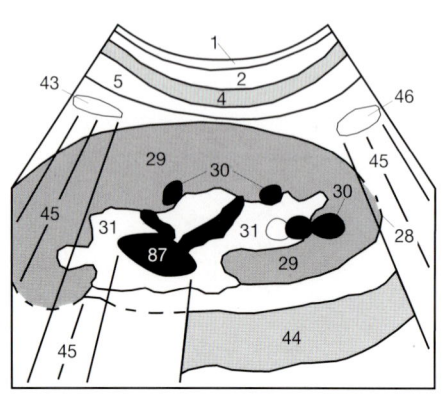

Fig. 40.1 b

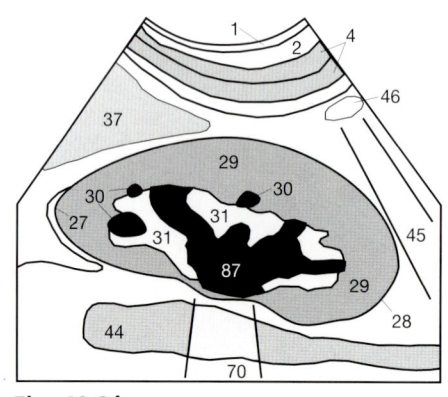

Fig. 40.2 b

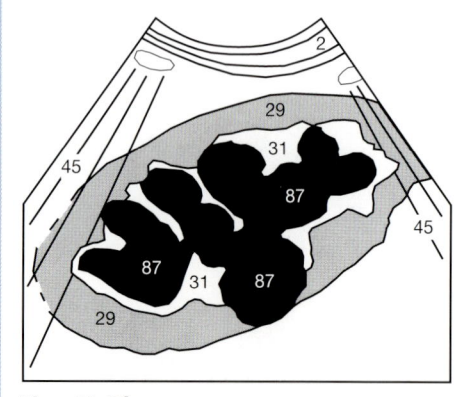

Fig. 40.3 b

5 Kidneys — Differential Diagnosis of Urinary Obstruction

Not every dilated renal pelvis (31) is indicative of obstructive uropathy. The developmental variant of an extrarenal pelvis was already mentioned on the preceding page. Furthermore, the renal hilum can show prominent vessels (25) (Fig. 41.1) that can be followed to the hypoechoic medullary pyramids (30) and might be mistaken for structures of the collecting system. These vessels generally appear rather delicate and lack the characteristic fullness found with an obstructed and dilated collecting system (compare Fig. 40.2).

If the findings are inconclusive, color Doppler sonography can easily determine whether these structures represent blood vessels containing rapidly flowing blood or the collecting system filled with essentially stationary urine. Blood vessels are seen as color-coded structures with the color depending on the direction and velocity of blood flow, while the barely moving urine in the collecting system remains black. The same principle of difference in relative flow can be employed to differentiate pelvic or peripelvic cysts (64), which do not require any therapy, from an obstructively dilated renal pelvis (87), which has to be expectantly observed or treated. Both conditions can, of course, concur (Fig. 41.2).

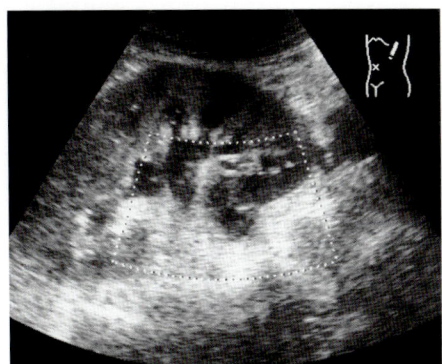

Fig. 41.1 a

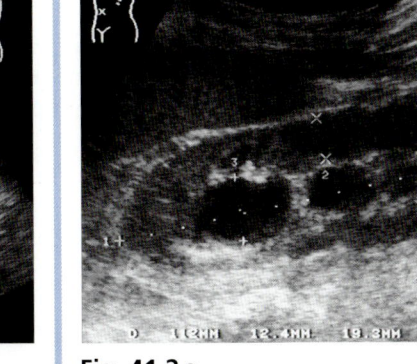

Fig. 41.2 a

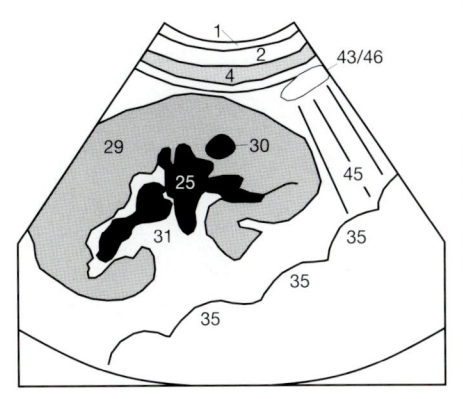

Fig. 41.1 b

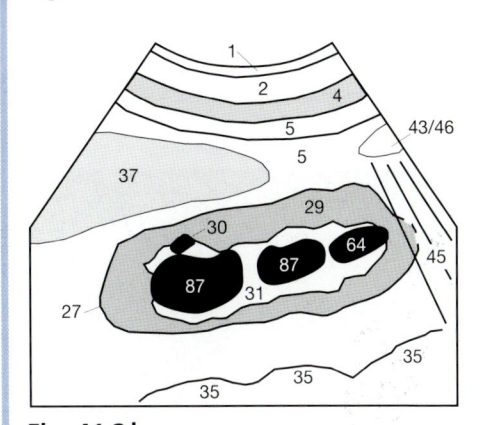

Fig. 41.2 b

Notes

5 Kidneys — Renal Stones and Infarcts

Detecting concrements in the kidney (nephrolithiasis) is more difficult than detecting stones in the gallbladder since the echogenic renal stones **(49)** are often located within the equally echogenic collecting system **(31)** **(Fig. 42.1)** and might not elicit any echogenicity that is discernible from its surrounding structures. Concrements in a dilated collecting system are a notable exception since they are easily revealed as echogenic structures within the echo-free urine. In the absence of any dilatation, it is of utmost importance to look for acoustic shadowing **(45)** caused by concrements or calcifications, such as is found in hyperparathyroidism.

Depending on its composition, a renal stone **(49)** can be either completely sound transmitting **(as seen in Fig. 42.1)** or so reflective that only its near surface is seen as echogenic cap **(Fig. 42.2)**. The differential diagnosis includes the arcuate arteries between the renal cortex and medullary pyramids (bright echoes *without* shadowing), vascular calcifications in diabetic patients, and calcified fibrotic residues following renal tuberculosis. Finally, papillary calcifications can occur after phenacetin abuse. Large staghorn calculi are difficult to diagnose if the distal acoustic shadowing is weak and its echogenicity mistaken for the central echogenic complex.

If renal concrements dislodge and migrate from the intrarenal collecting system into the ureter, they can, depending on their size, pass into the bladder without symptoms or with colics, or become lodged and cause ureteral obstruction. In addition to detecting obstructive uropathy, sonography can exclude other causes of abdominal pain, such as pancreatitis, colitis, and free fluid in the cul-de-sac.

Renal emboli or renal arterial stenosis can cause localized renal infarcts **(71)**, which, conforming to the vascular distribution, are broad-based at the renal surface and tapered toward the renal hilus. Sonographically, they are seen as triangular defects **(Fig. 42.3)** in the renal parenchyma **(29)**. The resultant scars are as echogenic as renal calculi but should not be mistaken for concrements on the basis of their form and localization.

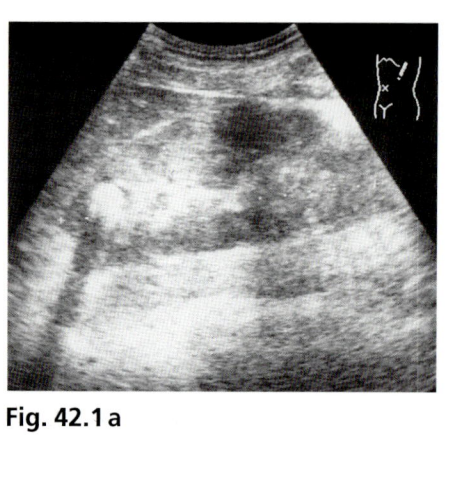

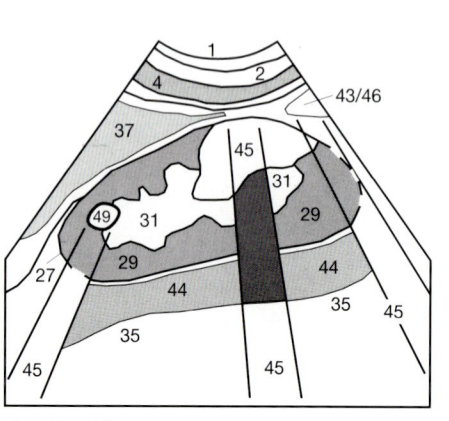

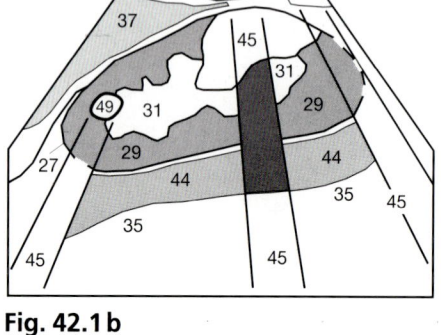

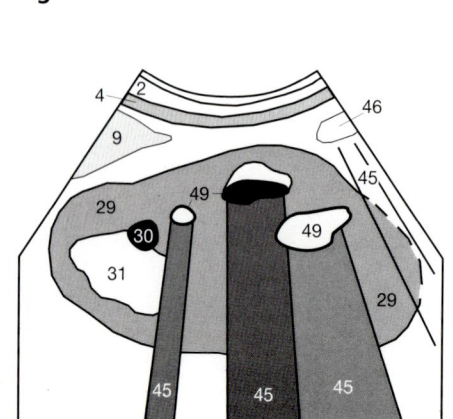

Fig. 42.1 a

Fig. 42.2 a

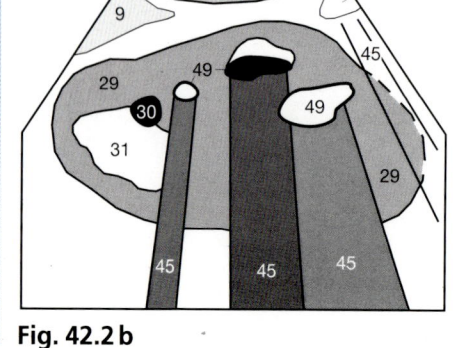

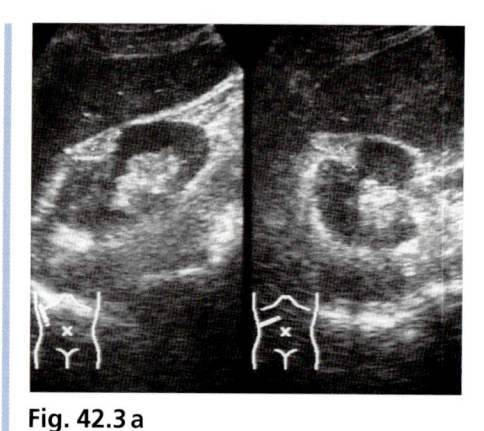

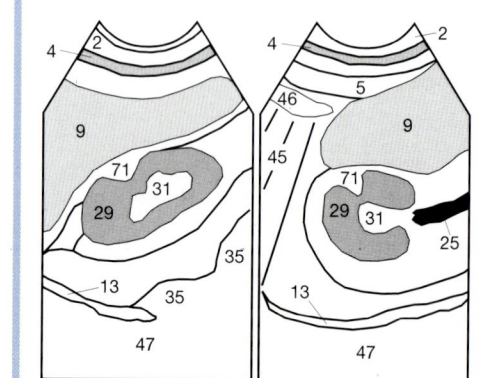

Fig. 42.3 a

Fig. 42.1 b

Fig. 42.2 b

Fig. 42.3 b

5 Kidneys — Renal Tumors

In contrast to fluid-filled cysts, solid renal tumors exhibit internal echoes and have only weak or no distal acoustic enhancement. Benign renal tumors (fibromas, adenomas, hemangiomas) are altogether rare with no uniform sonomorphology. Only the angiomyolipoma, a benign mixed tumor comprising vessels, muscular tissue, and fat, has in its early stage a characteristic sonographic presentation that separates it from a malignant process. A small angiomyolipoma (72) is as echogenic as the central echo complex and clearly demarcated (Fig. 43.1). With increasing size, angiomyolipomas become heterogeneous, rendering their differentiation from malignant tumors more difficult.

Small renal cell carcinomas (hypernephromas) are often iso-echoic with the remaining renal parenchyma (29). Only with further growth do the hypernephromas (54) become heterogeneous and space-occupying with bulging of the renal contour (Fig. 43.2). If a hypernephroma has been detected, the renal vein, related lymph-node-bearing sites, and contralateral kidney have to be carefully scrutinized for neoplastic changes. About 5% of renal cell carcinomas are bilateral, and advanced carcinomas can have vascular invasion with intravenous tumorous extension. If the tumor extends beyond the renal capsule and infiltrates the adjacent psoas muscle, the kidney loses its respiratory mobility.

The left adrenal gland lies anteromedial (not cranial) to the upper renal pole. The right adrenal gland extends posteriorly to the inferior vena cava. In adults, neither of the adrenal glands is visible, or only barely visible, in the perirenal fat. Hormone-producing adrenal tumors, such as an adenoma in Conn syndrome or hyperplasia in Cushing syndrome, are generally too small to be detectable sonographically. Only clinically manifest pheochromocytomas are often already several centimeters in size and can be sonographically detected in 90% of cases.

Sonography plays a more important role in the detection of adrenal metastases (54) (Fig. 43.3). Metastases are usually seen as hypoechoic lesions between the upper renal pole and spleen (37) or inferior hepatic surface, respectively, and must be differentiated from atypical renal cysts (Fig. 43.3). The hematogenous spread of metastases is attributed to the exquisite vascularity of the adrenal glands and can be found with bronchogenic carcinomas as well as with carcinomas of the breast and kidney. Whether or not a suprarenal space-occupying lesion is malignant cannot be deduced from the lesion's echogenicity. Before proceeding to a needle biopsy, a pheochromocytoma must be excluded to avoid precipitating a hypertensive crisis.

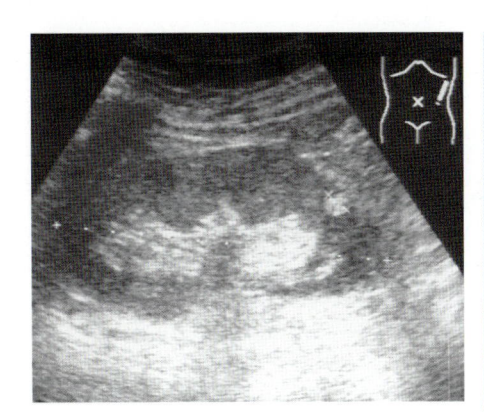

Fig. 43.1 a

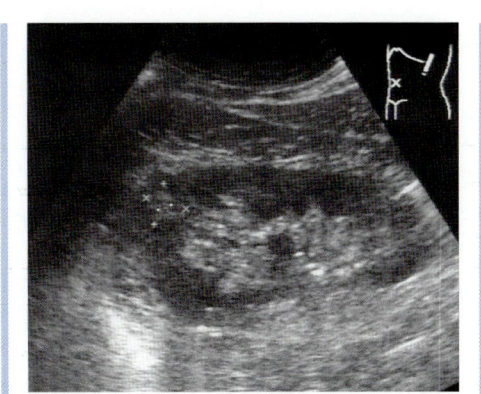

Fig. 43.2 a

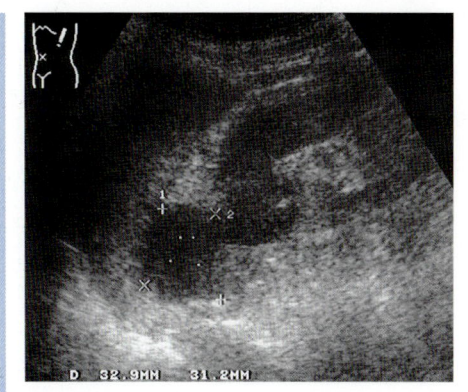

Fig. 43.3 a

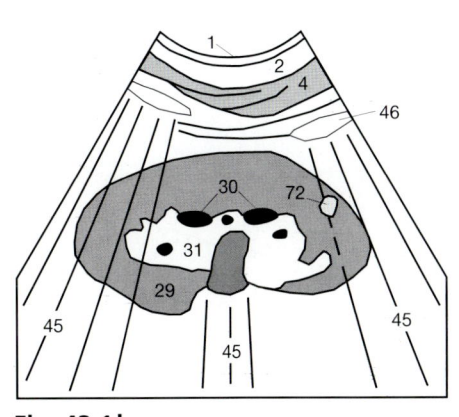

Fig. 43.1 b

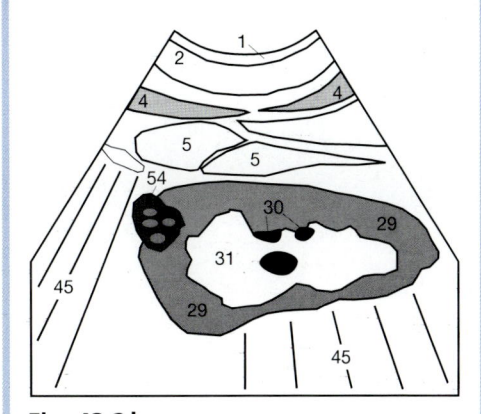

Fig. 43.2 b

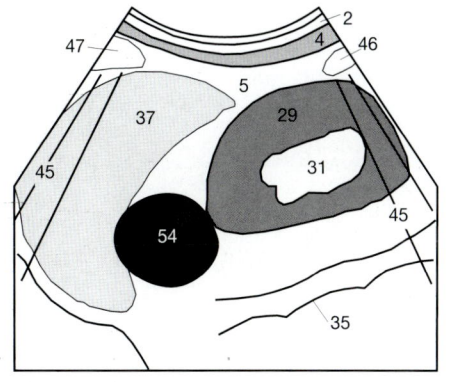

Fig. 43.3 b

5 Kidneys — Renal Transplant: Normal Findings

Renal transplants can be in either of the iliac fossa and are connected to the iliac vessels. Like the orthotopic kidneys, they are sonographically examined in two projections **(Fig. 44.1)**, but the transducer is placed over the lateral aspect of the lower abdomen. No interfering intestinal air is present because of the superficial position of the transplanted kidney just beneath the anterior abdominal wall.

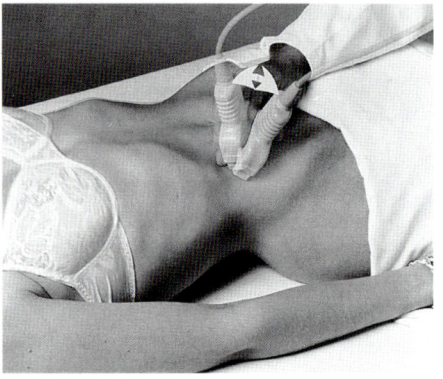

Fig. 44.1 a

Fig. 44.1 b

It is crucial to detect a rejection or other complications early (compare p. 45). It is normal for a renal transplant to show an often permanent increase in size by up to 20% after surgery. In comparison with the native kidneys, its cortex **(29)** appears wider **(Fig. 44.2)** and the parenchymal echogenicity can increase so that the medullary pyramids **(30)** become better demarcated. Progressive inflammatory infiltration must be excluded by serial sonographic studies, which should be obtained at short intervals during the immediate postoperative period. A prominent renal pelvis or a slightly distended (first degree) collecting system **(compare Figs. 40.1, 40.2)** might be observed without requiring intervention because of functional impairment of the renal transplant. The urinary distention should be documented and measured in cross section **(Fig. 44.3)** to avoid missing on subsequent studies any progression that might require therapeutic intervention.

The renal transplant should be further evaluated for the distinctness of its outline and its interface between the parenchyma **(29)** and collecting system **(31)**. An indistinct PP-interface or a slight increase in volume can be warning signs of the onset of rejection. To allow a valid comparison, reproducible longitudinal and transverse diameters should be selected for measurements and documentation (compare p. 45). After transplantation, the immunosuppressive medications can gradually be reduced and the intervals between the sonographic studies extended.

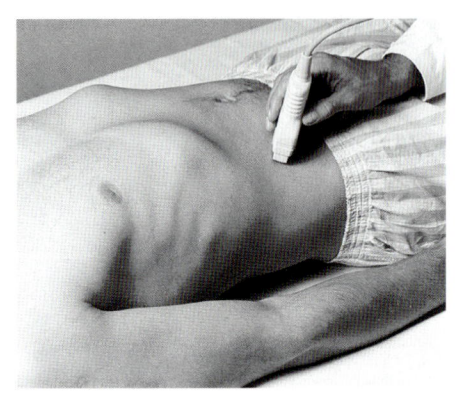

Fig. 44.2 a

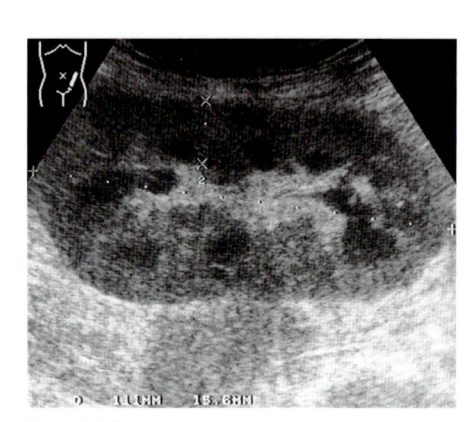

Fig. 44.2 b

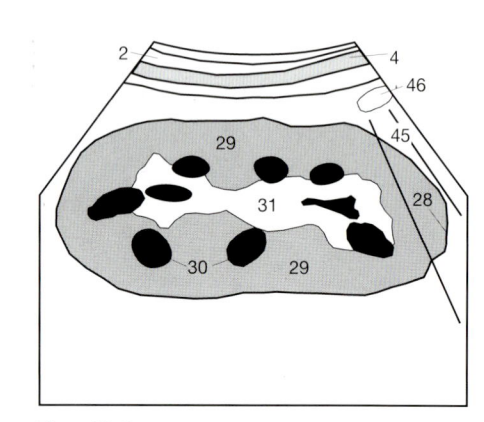

Fig. 44.2 c

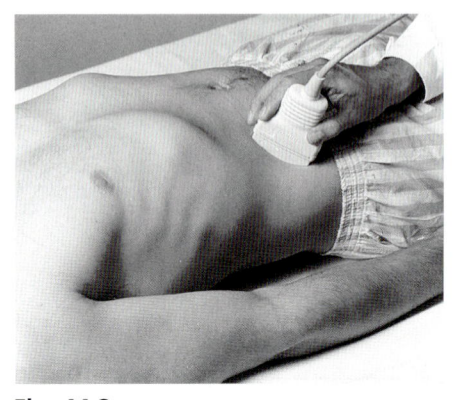

Fig. 44.3 a

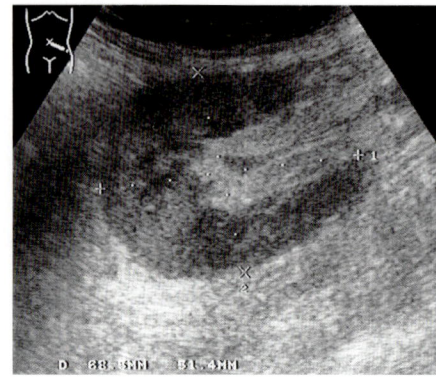

Fig. 44.3 b

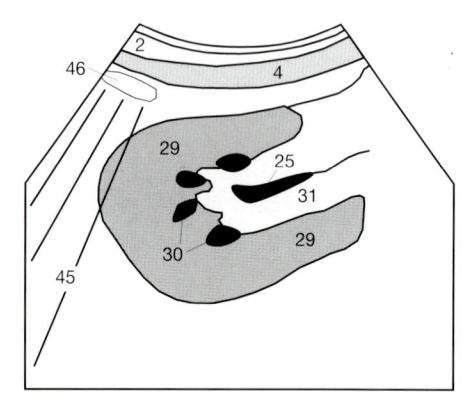

Fig. 44.3 c

5 Kidneys — Renal Transplant

For an accurate assessment of its size, the renal transplant has to be visualized longitudinally first **(Fig. 45.1b)** and the position of the transducer then adjusted until the maximal length comes into view. The diagram **(Fig. 45.1a)** illustrates a line too far lateral (dotted line) that would measure a spuriously short distance. To get to the "true" longitudinal dimension (d_L) the transducer has to be tilted along the straight arrows.

Thereafter, the transducer is slightly turned **(Fig. 45.1c)** until there is no longer angulation along the curved arrow **(Fig. 45.1a)**. This two-step approach to guiding the transducer should assure that the length documented is not too short, which could lead to a spurious increase in the calculated volume (simplified volume formula: vol = A x B x C x 0.5) on follow-up examinations.

A lymphocele **(73)** can develop as a complication after renal transplant surgery **(Fig. 45.2)** and is usually found between the lower pole of the renal transplant and the urinary bladder **(38)**, but can be anywhere adjacent to the transplant. Urinary obstruction **(87)** is an equally frequent complication and, depending on its severity, might require temporary stent drainage **(59)** **(Figs. 45.3, 45.4)** to prevent damage of the renal parenchyma **(29)**. Measuring the RI of the supplying renal vessel by Doppler sonography provides additional information concerning the condition of the renal transplant.

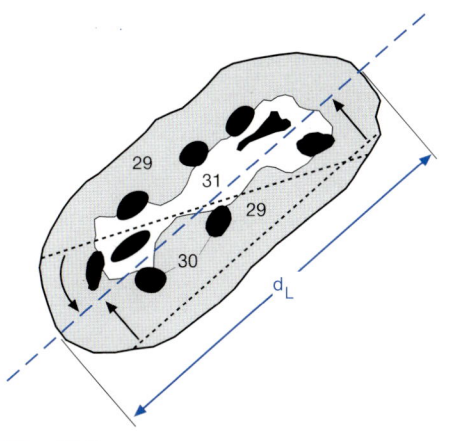

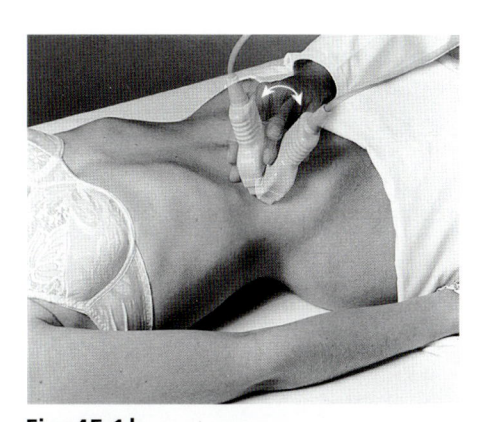

Fig. 45.1 a

Fig. 45.1 b

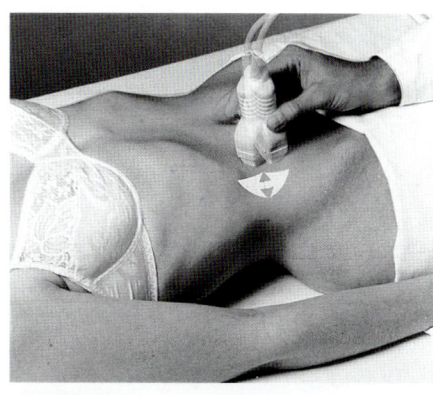

Fig. 45.1 c

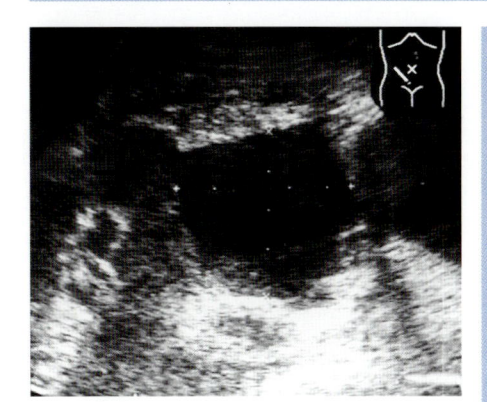

Fig. 45.2 a

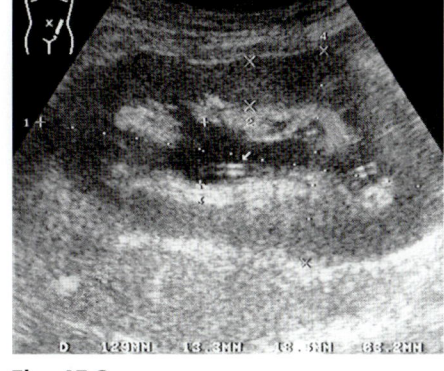

Fig. 45.3 a

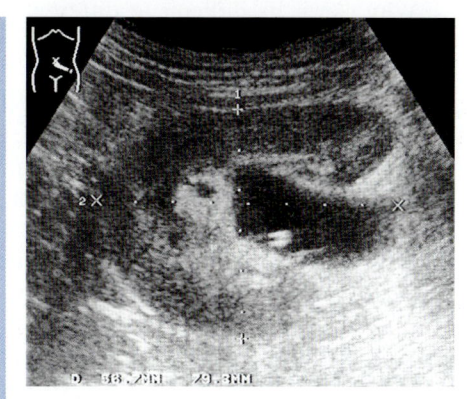

Fig. 45.4 a

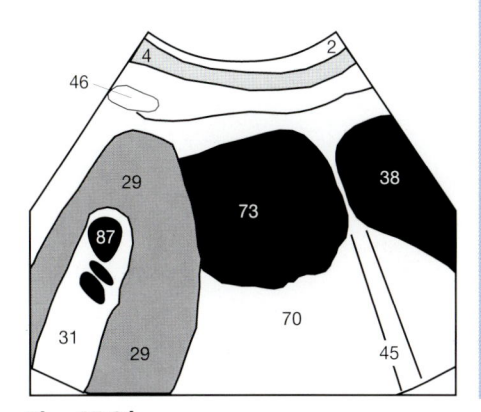

Fig. 45.2 b

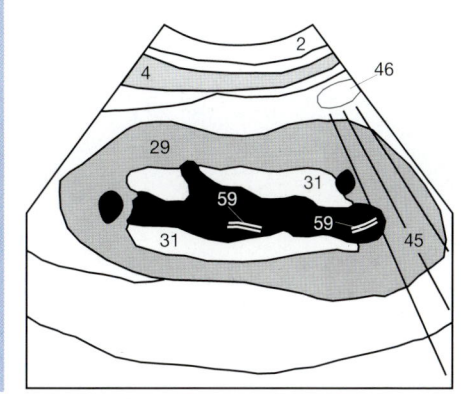

Fig. 45.3 b

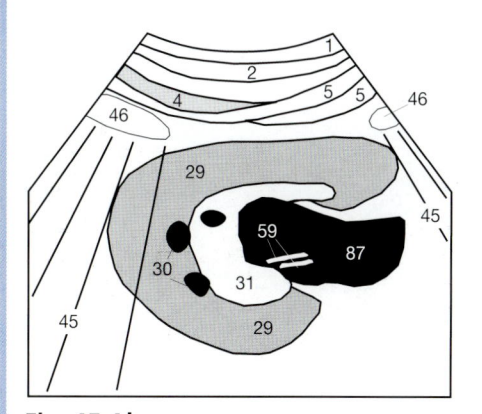

Fig. 45.4 b

5 Kidneys — Quiz for Self-Assessment

It is the goal of this workbook to provide factual knowledge and to facilitate memorization by means of most effective teaching strategies. This should facilitate immediate and rapid recall from memory whenever necessary at a later time. Empirically, it has been shown that beginners in sonography become faster and better oriented with the three-dimensional abdominal space if they are able to sketch the few standard orientations from memory. Do not get annoyed at the following questions: there are no better teaching methods that relate new material in a shorter period of time.

1 From memory, draw a typical transverse section of the right kidney at the level of its hilum, including its position relative to the liver and inferior vena cava. How would the corresponding body marker look? Compare your drawing with the diagram shown on page 37 (the body marker has been left out intentionally).

2 Try, by means of a sketch, to characterize the different shapes of the normal kidney, the kidney with prominent vessels, and the kidney with mild to severe (grade I to grade III) dilatation. Discuss with a fellow trainee the criteria that differentiate these five possibilities. It is not the other trainee's lack of comprehension but your fault if your he or she cannot reconstruct the findings you describe. Compare your sketches afterwards with **Figures 37.2c, 41.1b, 40.2b, and 40.3b**.

3 How would you recognize a nephrolithiasis? What possible underlying conditions are there? By consulting a textbook, try to list the possible causes of hematuria (blood in the urine).

4 List the sonographic criteria of a renal angiomyolipoma. Why can it be difficult to differentiate its findings from other renal tumors?

5 Write down the normal values for the longitudinal and transverse diameters of the kidneys, for the width of the renal parenchyma, and for the respiratory mobility. Compare your values with those listed on page 37.

6 Review carefully the sonographic images provided and write down next to each image all visualized organs and muscles as well as your diagnosis, including your reasons for arriving at this diagnosis. After you are done, compare your results with the answers given on page 77.

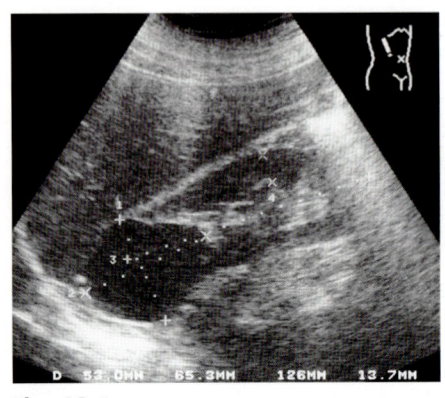

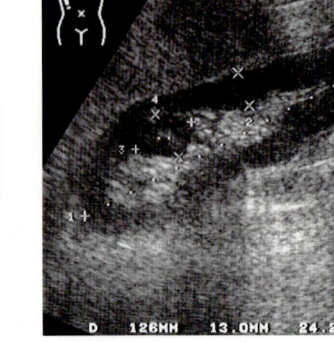

Fig. 46.1

Fig. 46.2

6 Spleen

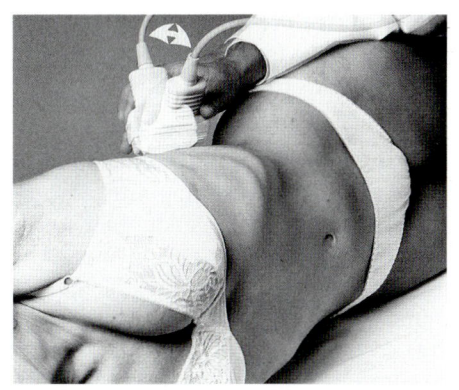

Normal Findings

Fig. 47.1

The spleen is visualized in the right lateral decubitus position with the patient taking a deep breath (Fig. 47.2a). The transducer is placed parallel to the intercostal space to avoid interfering acoustic shadows (45) that arise from the ribs. The spleen is carefully scrutinized from the diaphragmatic dome (13) to the level of its hilar vessels (20) (Fig. 47.1).

Frequently, visualization of the spleen is compromised by air in the left lung (47) or in an adjacent intestinal loop (43). Normal splenic measurements are 4 × 7 × 11 cm ("4711" rule), whereby the maximum diameter measured in this visualized plane between hilum and diaphragmatic surface of the spleen should be 4 cm.

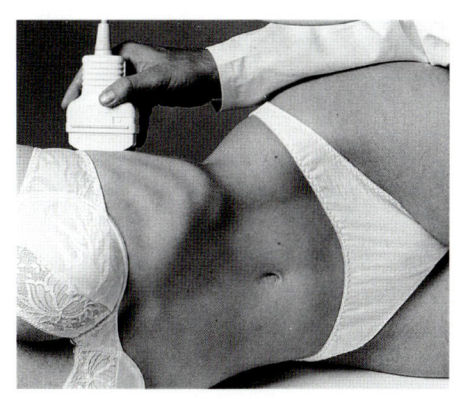

Fig. 47.2 a

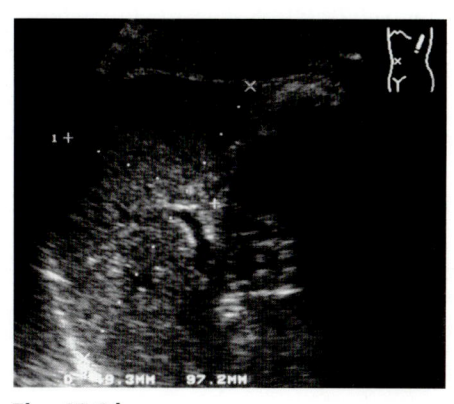

Fig. 47.2 b

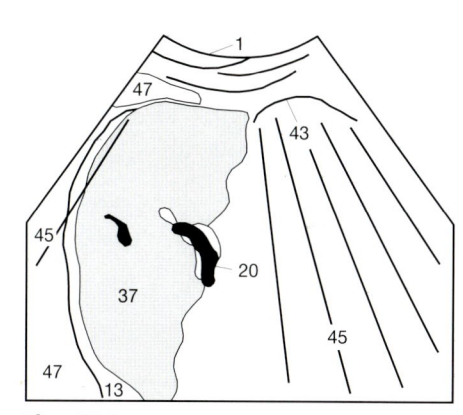

Fig. 47.2 c

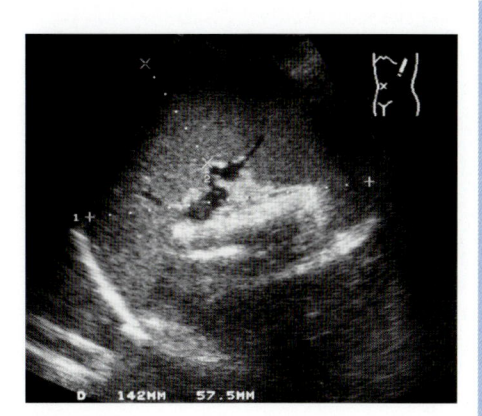

Fig. 47.3 a

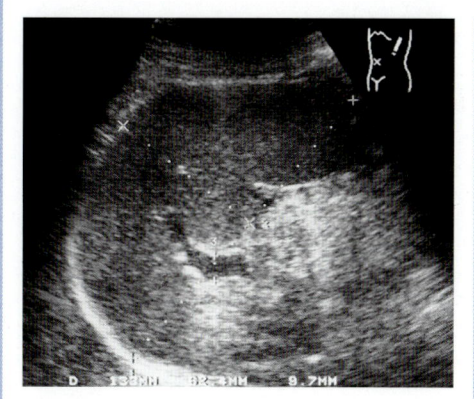

Fig. 47.4 a

Suggestion: If the inspiration is too deep, the lung (47) extends inferiorly into the diaphragmatic angle and obscures the subdiaphragmatic portion of the spleen (Fig. 47.3). In this situation, the "curtain trick" should be tried by asking the patient to exhale *slowly* following maximal inspiration until the spleen becomes visible (Fig. 47.4). Like a curtain, the lung frequently recedes before the spleen (37) moves back upward. During this asynchronous rate of retraction, the moment has to be watched for when the acoustic shadows (45) from the lung no longer interfere with visualization of the spleen. At that point, the patient has to be asked to hold his or her breath.

Occasionally, the spleen is better seen in the supine than in the right lateral decubitus position.

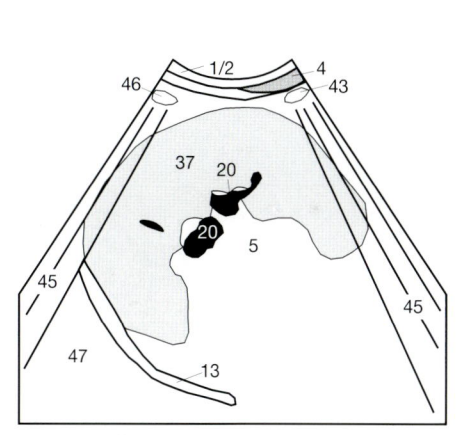

Fig. 47.3 b

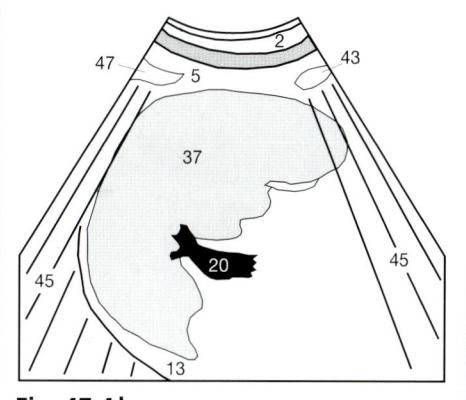

Fig. 47.4 b

6 Spleen

Diffuse Splenomegaly

Many conditions are associated with diffuse enlargement of the spleen, and the differential diagnosis does not only include portal hypertension **(Fig. 48.2)** secondary to hepatic cirrhosis but also viral infections, such as mononucleosis. Furthermore, all diseases causing an increased turnover of erythrocytes, such as hemolytic anemia and polycythemia vera, can produce a splenomegaly **(Fig. 48.3)**.

Splenomegaly typically accompanies systemic hematologic diseases, such as acute or chronic leukemia (**Fig. 48.1** in CLL), but can be found in rheumatic, immunologic, and storage diseases. Not every splenomegaly is of pathologic relevance since many diseases heal by leaving behind a mild to moderate splenomegaly, for instance mononucleosis. The enlargement of the spleen **(37)** begins with a rounding of its normal crescentic configuration **(Fig. 47.2)** and can progress to the so-called "giant spleen." The massively enlarged spleen can touch the left hepatic lobe and this is referred to as "kissing phenomenon." Occasionally, an accessory spleen can reach a considerable size. Accessory spleens **(86)** **(Fig. 48.1)** are generally located at the splenic hilum or adjacent to the lower splenic pole and cannot always be differentiated from enlarged lymph nodes **(55)** **(Fig. 48.3)**.

Suggestions: If the sonographic examination of the abdomen reveals a splenomegaly, a systemic hematologic condition must be considered and all node-bearing areas of the abdomen should be explored for any lymphadenopathy (see pp. 14 and 21). Furthermore, portal hypertension should be excluded by measuring the luminal diameter of the splenic vein **(20)**, portal vein, and superior mesenteric vein and by searching for portocaval collaterals. The size of the spleen should be measured accurately. Only by having a baseline measurement of the splenic size can subsequent examinations determine any interval growth. Questions that subsequent examinations might address, such as possible interval growth during therapy, should already be kept in mind during the initial examination. Neither size nor echogenicity of the spleen allows any inference as to the nature of the underlying condition.

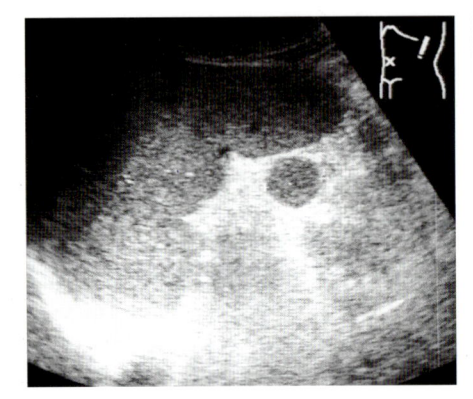

Fig. 48.1 a

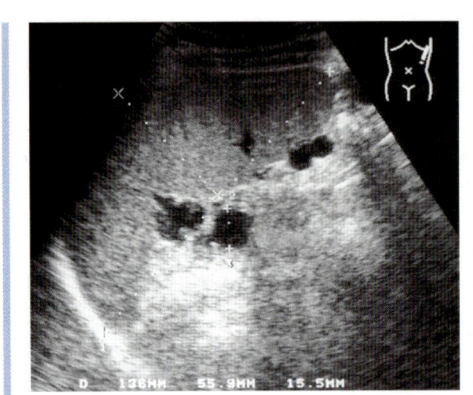

Fig. 48.2 a

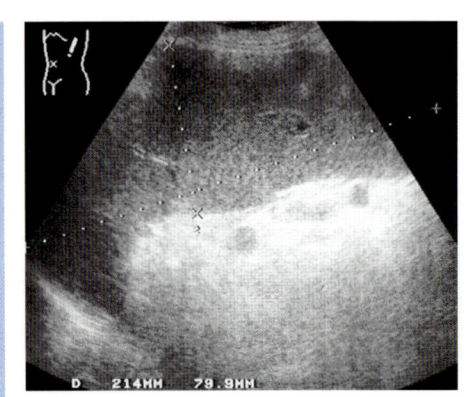

Fig. 48.3 a

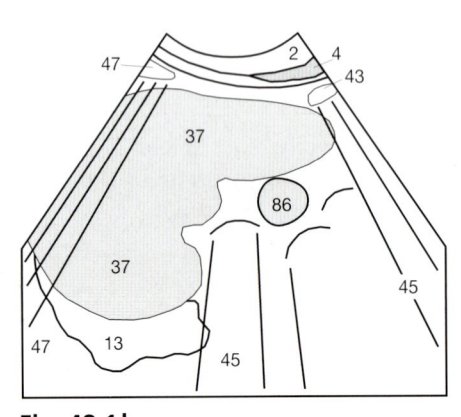

Fig. 48.1 b

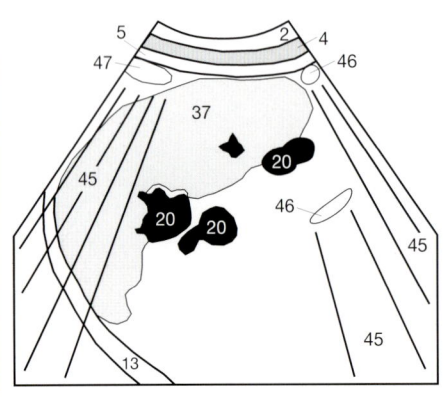

Fig. 48.2 b

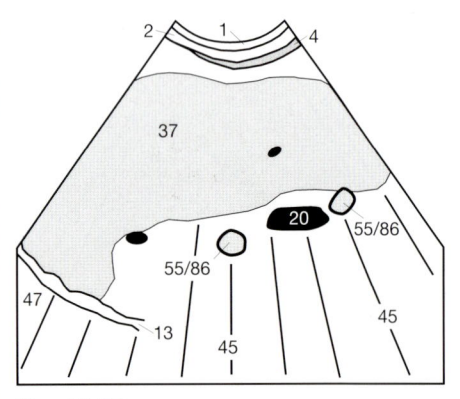

Fig. 48.3 b

6 Spleen

Focal Splenic Changes

Areas that are hypoechoic in relation to the remaining splenic parenchyma include as possible causes all focal lymphomatous infiltrations. In non-Hodgkin lymphoma, these lymphomatous infiltrations can be localized as well as diffuse throughout the spleen giving it a heterogeneous appearance. Congenital (dysontogenetic) splenic cysts are rather uncommon and do not differ sonographically from hepatic cysts **(64) (Fig. 29.1)**, thus they are not illustrated again here. Acquired splenic cysts frequently develop after trauma or infarcts. As is true for hepatic cysts, internal septations suggest a parasitic origin **(compare Fig. 30.3)**.

Recognizing a splenic hematoma **(Fig. 49.2)** might be difficult since a fresh hemorrhage can be iso-echoic with the surrounding splenic parenchyma **(37)**. In general, the echogenicity of the extravasated blood decreases within a few days, and subacute or old hematomas **(50)** are usually well visualized as hypoechoic space-occupying lesions. A parenchymal laceration without a capsular tear can produce an initially unrecognized subcapsular hematoma. The risk of such a hematoma is a delayed tear of the splenic capsule, which releases the tamponaded hematoma and causes free bleeding into the abdominal cavity. More than 50% of these so-called "delayed" splenic ruptures occur within 1 week after the trauma, and it is advisable during this interval at least to perform serial follow-up studies.

Finally, the spleen can exhibit echogenic foci. They could represent splenic hemangiomas, which are rare, or calcified granulomas, which are rather common and usually found with tuberculosis or histoplasmosis. Splenic calcifications can also accompany cirrhosis. A spleen harboring multiple echogenic foci **(53)** has been called the „star-sky spleen" **(Fig. 49.3)**. Splenic abscesses and splenic metastases, which are rare, can have a rather varied sonomorphology, in part depending on their duration and underlying cause. There are no simple reliable differential diagnostic criteria, and consultation of reference textbooks is recommended. Splenic infarcts **(71)** can be observed in splenomegaly with compromised vascular supply **(Fig. 49.1)**.

Suggestion: Patients with acute abdominal and thoracic trauma should be searched for free fluid in the cul-de-sac and below the diaphragm **(13)** as well as around the spleen and liver. Carefully scrutinize the spleen for a double contour along its capsule (subcapsular hematoma?) and for a heterogeneous echo pattern of its parenchyma, to avoid overlooking a possible splenic rupture.

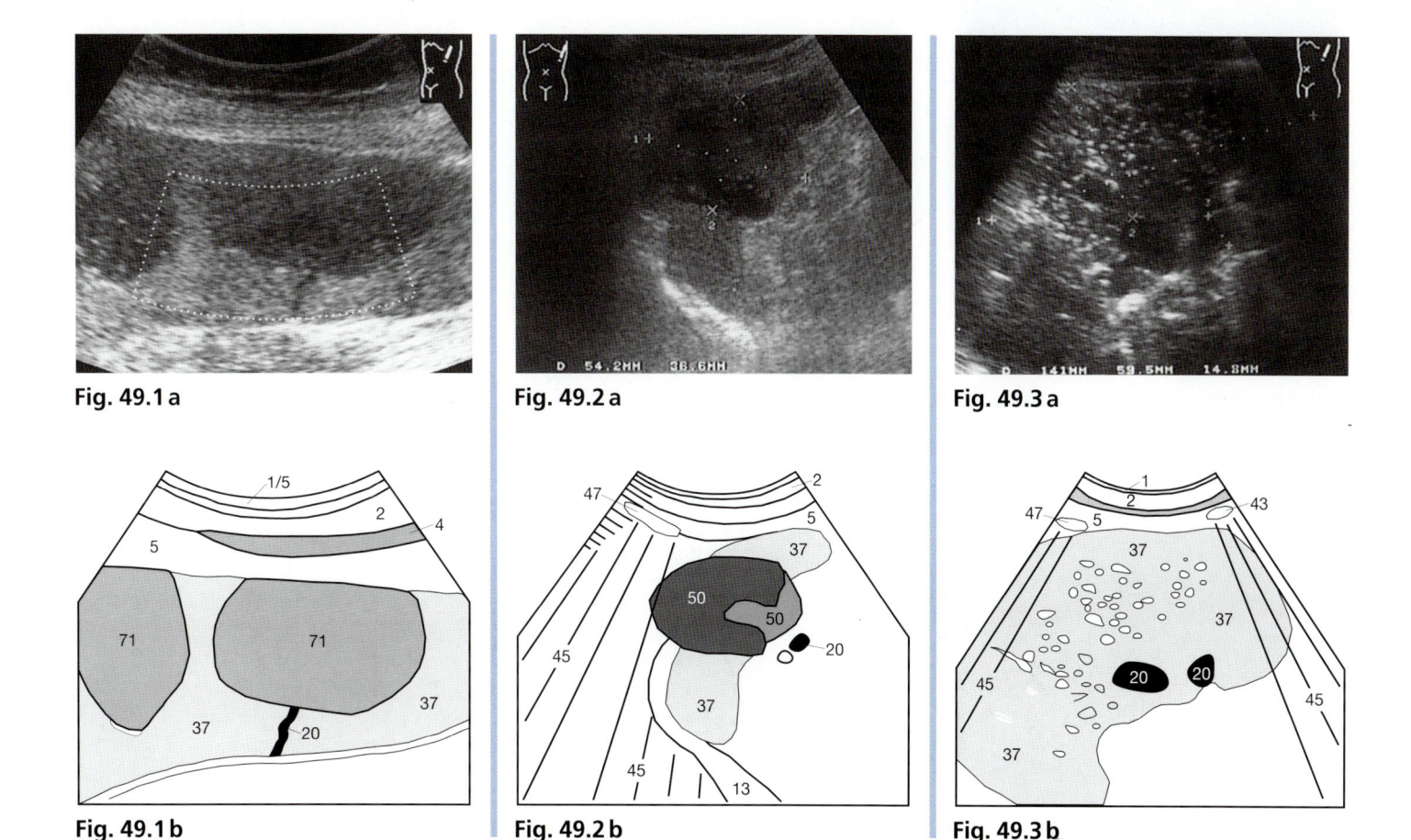

Fig. 49.1 a

Fig. 49.2 a

Fig. 49.3 a

Fig. 49.1 b

Fig. 49.2 b

Fig. 49.3 b

6 Spleen — Quiz for Self-Assessment

The material about the spleen presented in the preceding three pages should have prepared you to answer the following questions. The answers to questions 1 to 4 are contained in the text, and the answer to question 5 is found on page 77.

1 What are the diameters (maximal values) of a normal spleen?

2 What structure frequently superimposes air over the spleen and how can this be remedied?

3 What must the examiner search for in patients who have sustained a blunt abdominal trauma?

4 How should the examination be extended if a splenomegaly is found?

5 Examine this image of a clinical case step by step:
— What sonographic section is it?
— What organ is primarily shown?
— What other structures can be seen?
— Is the parenchymal pattern normal?
— If the answer is negative, how can the changes be described?
— Try to give a differential diagnosis.

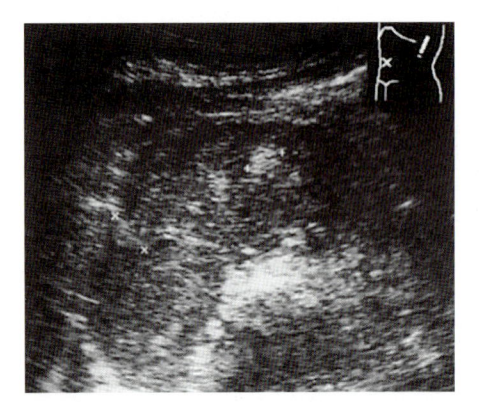

Fig. 50.1

Notes

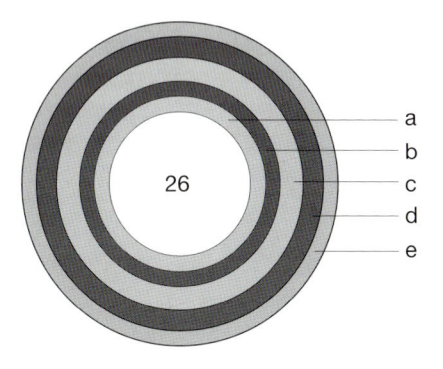

7 GI Tract — Stomach

The normal mural layers of the GI tract can be seen in **Figure 51.1**. Abdominal sonography at best shows three (c, d, e) of the five mural layers. The transducer is placed over the left upper quadrant of the abdomen **(Fig. 51.2 a)**. In the NPO patient, the mural layers **(74)** of the gastric antrum **(26)** can be seen behind the liver **(9)** and directly in front of the pancreas **(33)** **(Figs. 51.2 b, c)**. Air shadowing **(45)** precludes a reliable evaluation in patients who have meteorism or are postprandial. If the stomach is markedly distended **(Fig. 51.3)**, wall-based tumors **(54)** or muscular thickening as manifestation of pyloric hypertrophy **(Figs. 51.4, 51.5)** must be looked for.

Depending on its state of contraction, the gastric wall should measure 5–7 mm and the hypoechoic lamina muscularis by itself not more than 5 mm. Any suspicious gastric lesions should be further evaluated by gastroscopy or radiography.

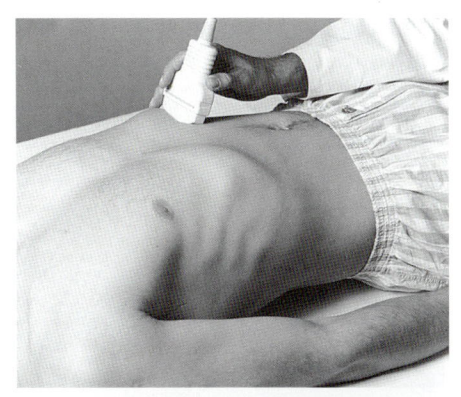

The endosonographic presentation of the mural layers of the GI tract:
Gastric lumen (26)
Strongly echogenic mucosal interface (a)
Weakly echogenic mucosa (b)
Strongly echogenic submucosa (c)
Weakly echogenic lamina muscularis (d)
Strongly echogenic serosa interface (e)

Fig. 51.1

Fig. 51.2 a

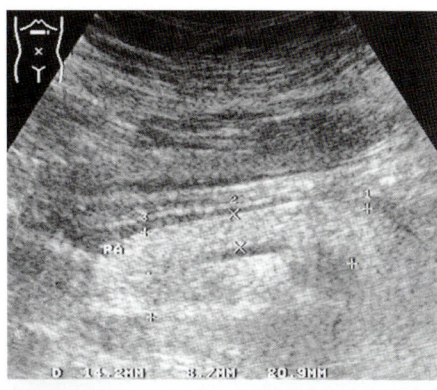

Fig. 51.2 b

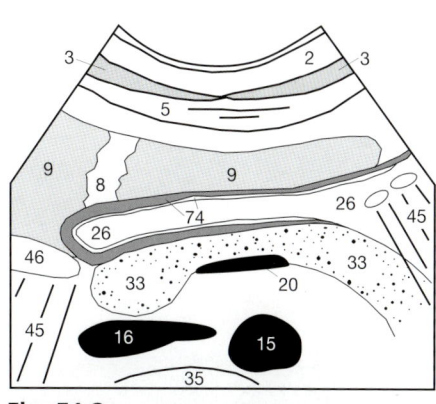

Fig. 51.2 c

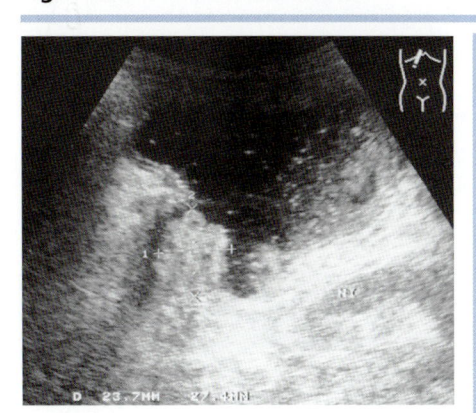

Fig. 51.3 a

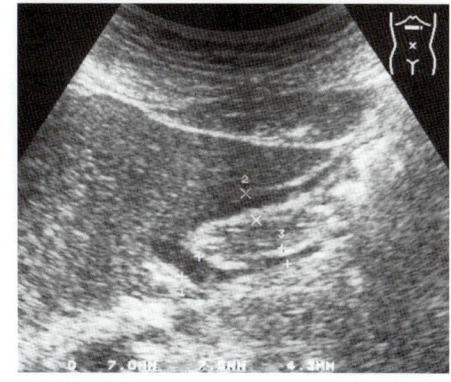

Fig. 51.4 a

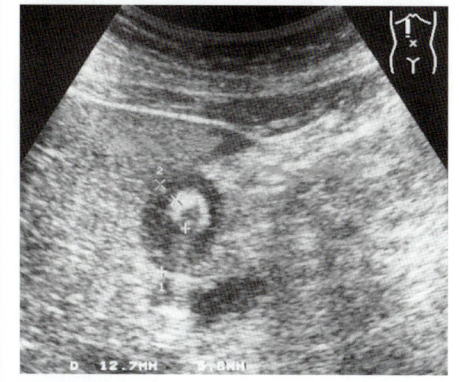

Fig. 51.5 a

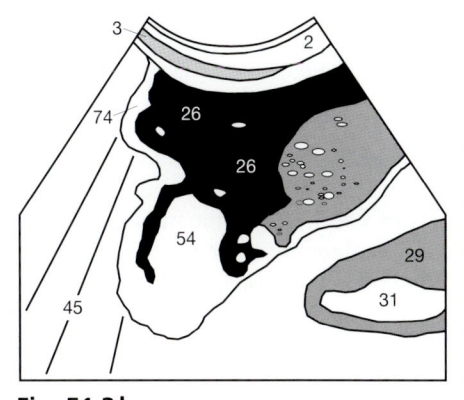

Fig. 51.3 b

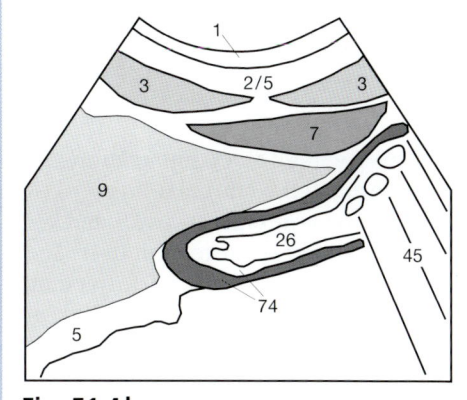

Fig. 51.4 b

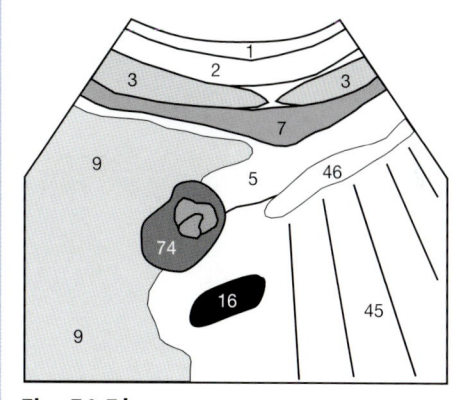

Fig. 51.5 b

7 GI Tract | Colon

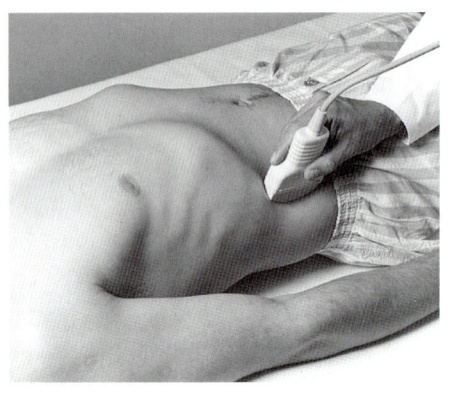

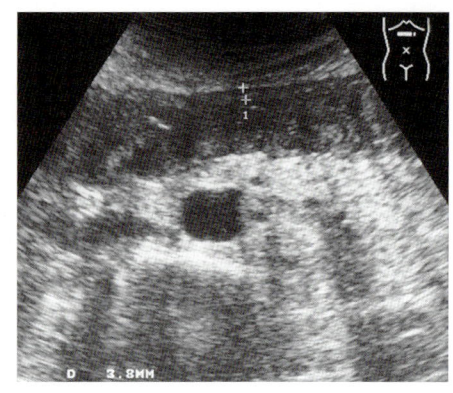

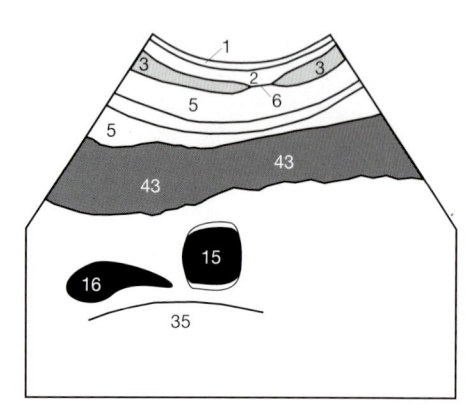

Fig. 52.1 a

Fig. 52.1 b

Fig. 52.1 c

The ascending colon can be seen in the lateral sagittal section **(Fig. 52.1 a)**. In most cases, air in the colon precludes visualization of its lumen. Large amounts of retained fecal matter (coprostasis) can occasionally be found in the colon of old patients. A transverse colon **(43)** without any evidence of inflammatory mural thickening (transverse section of the upper abdomen) is shown in **Figures 52.1 b and c**. This contrasts with the thickened wall **(74)** found in ulcerative colitis or ischemia (e.g. due to mesenteric artery infarction or mesenteric vein thrombosis), as seen in a case of colitis **(Fig. 52.2)** in which the descending colon exhibits strikingly thickened haustral indentations.

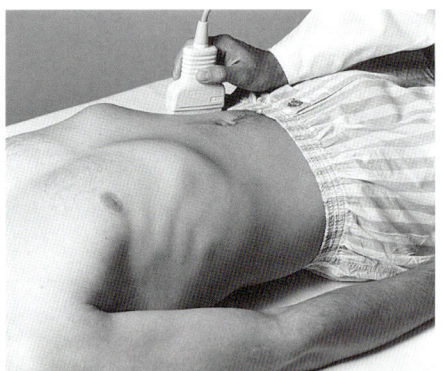

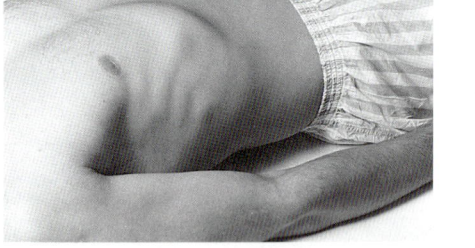

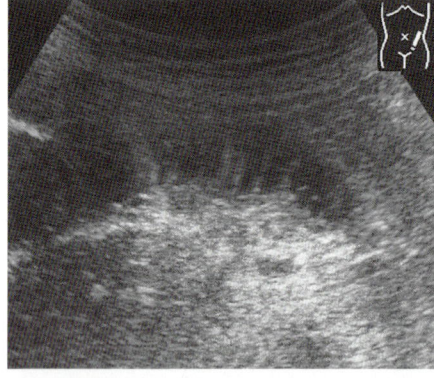

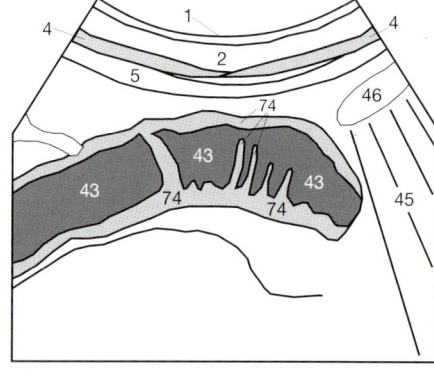

Fig. 52.2 a

Fig. 52.2 b

Fig. 52.2 c

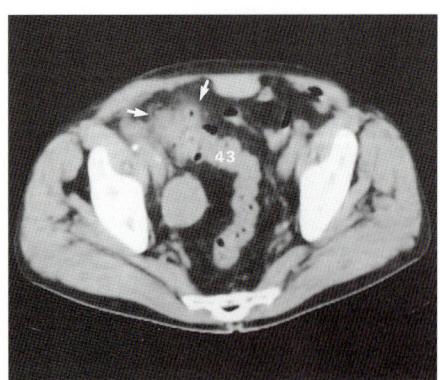

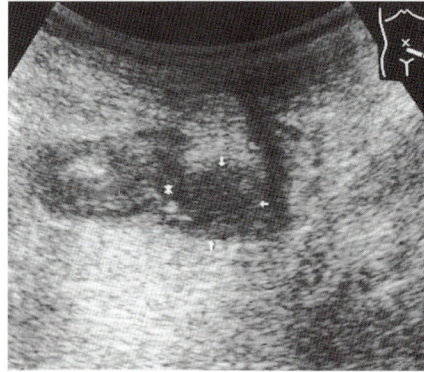

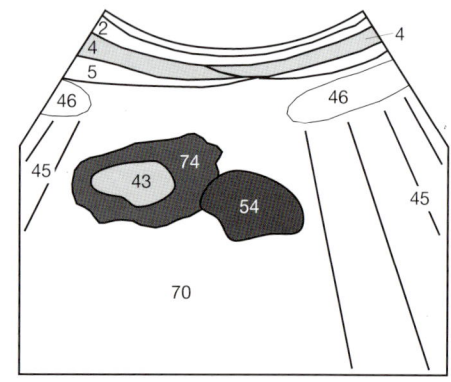

Fig. 52.3 a

Fig. 52.3 b

Fig. 52.3 c

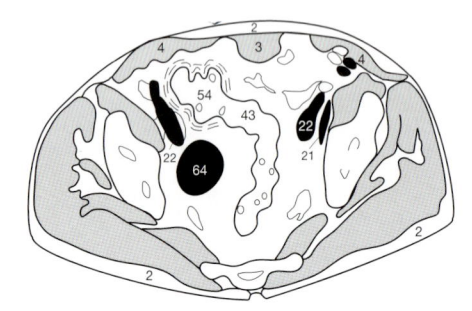

Fig. 52.3 d

Diverticulitis is a complication of diverticulosis coli (sac–like mucosal projections through the muscular layers of the colonic wall). The neck of the diverticulum (*), as shown in **Figures 52.3 b and c**, connects the normal colonic lumen **(43)** and the hypoechoic diverticulum **(54)**. The associated edema of the colonic wall **(74)** is demonstrated by the CT performed on the same patient **(Figs. 52.3 a, d)**. The rectosigmoid junction is still well demarcated from the hypodense fatty tissue (black), while the colonic wall is indistinct in outline in the immediate proximity of the diverticula **(54)** due to inflammatory obliteration and thickening of the adjacent fatty tissue.

7 GI Tract — Small Bowel

Because of air in the intestinal lumen, the sonographic evaluation of small bowel loops **(46)** is often limited or not possible at all. However, the intraluminal air frequently decreases when it is surrounded by inflammatory wall thickening or can be reduced by graded (!) compression applied to the transducer.

Crohn disease frequently presents as terminal ileitis **(Fig. 53.1)**. The edematous wall thickening **(74)** confined to this segment is easily separable from adjacent uninvolved loops **(46)**. In more advanced stages **(Fig. 53.2)**, the intestinal wall **(74)** becomes massively thickened and can resemble the sonographic findings of intestinal invagination. On cross sections, the thickened, edematous walls of intestinal loops can be compared to a concentric lamellation of a "target." The examiner should always look for adjacent fistular tracts or abscesses as well as for free abdominal fluid in the cul-de-sac.

The mesenteric roots of individual small bowel loops are normally not identified, but can be delineated in the presence of extensive lymphadenopathy or massive ascites **(68)**. The small bowel loop seen in cross section **(46)** floats within ascitic fluid **(Fig. 53.3)** that is devoid of internal echoes except for reverberation artifacts from the anterior abdominal wall **(2, 3)** (compare p. 10). Lymphomatous infiltration of the small bowel often leads to long segments of hypoechoic wall thickening and is primarily observed in immunocompromised patients.

High frequency transducers (> 5 MHz) can add information in selected cases if used, for instance, intraoperatively to exclude mesenteric lymphadenopathy. If a tender appendix shows no peristalsis, has reduced or no compressibility, and measures more than 6 mm in diameter, it fulfills the criteria of acute appendicitis. Sonography has the advantage of allowing real time evaluation of intestinal peristalsis, easily revealing aperistalsis (atony) or prestenotic hyperperistalsis. Though it is often necessary to proceed with other imaging modalities (endoscopy, endosonography, conventional radiology, CT) because of acoustic shadowing **(45)** by intestinal air that limits the sonographic evaluation of the small bowel, sonography can still make a contribution if properly targeted in selected cases.

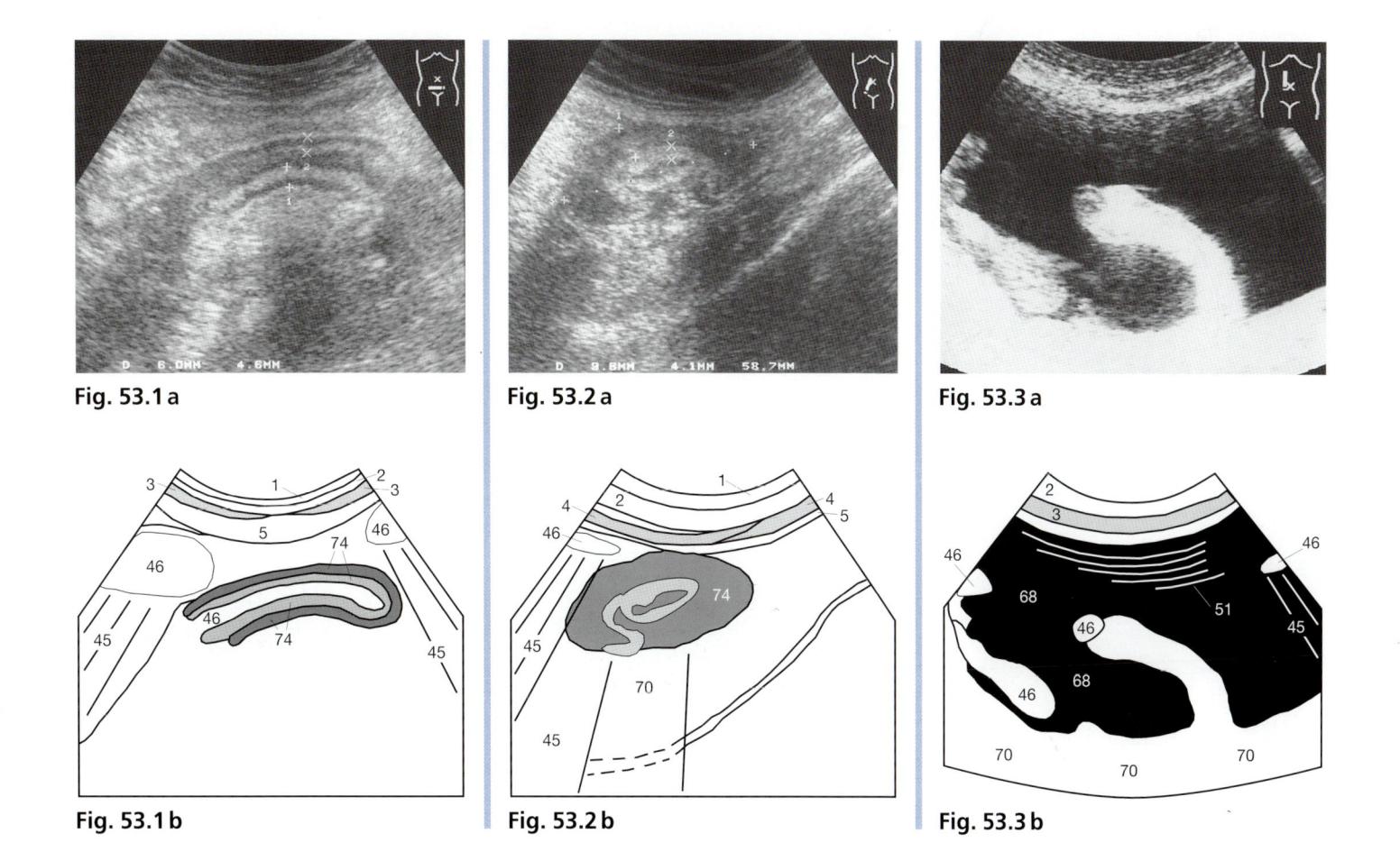

Fig. 53.1 a

Fig. 53.2 a

Fig. 53.3 a

Fig. 53.1 b

Fig. 53.2 b

Fig. 53.3 b

8 Urinary Bladder

Normal Findings, Volume Measurements

The urinary bladder is systematically screened in suprapubic transverse **(Fig. 54.1 a)** and sagittal sections **(Fig. 54.1 b)** when it is full, usually achieved after the intake of a large amount of fluid.

A representative transverse section **(Fig. 54.2)** shows the normal bladder **(38)** in the shape of a rounded rectangle behind the rectus muscles **(3)** and in front of and above the rectum **(43)**.

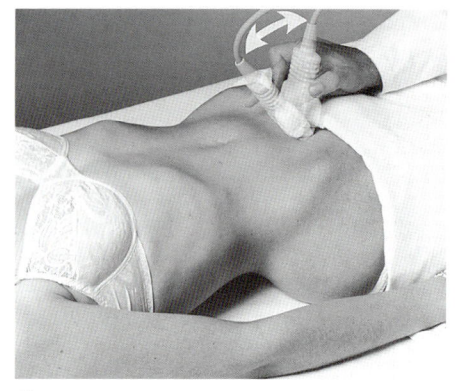

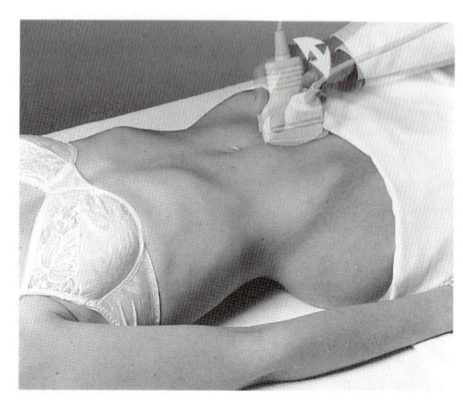

Fig. 54.1 a

Fig. 54.1 b

The longitudinal section delineates the bladder more as a triangle **(Fig. 54.3)**, with the prostate gland **(42)** and vagina, respectively, seen below the bladder (compare **Fig. 58.1**).

If voiding difficulties due to a neurogenic bladder or prostatic hypertrophy **(Figs. 56.2, 56.3)** are suspected, the postvoid residual should be calculated by measuring the maximum transverse and sagittal diameters of the bladder after the patient has voided **(Fig. 54.2 b)**. Thereafter, the transducer is turned 90° and angled inferiorly **(Fig. 54.3 a)** to measure the craniocaudal diameter (horizontally displayed on the image) without interfering acoustic shadowing **(45)** of the pubic symphysis **(48)** **(Fig. 54.3 b)**.

Using the simplified volume formula (vol$_{ub}$ = A x B x C x 0.5), the postvoid residual (ml) can be calculated by dividing the product of the three diameters by two.

Find out which diameter in the case shown in **Figure 54.3 b** has been incidentally measured twice?

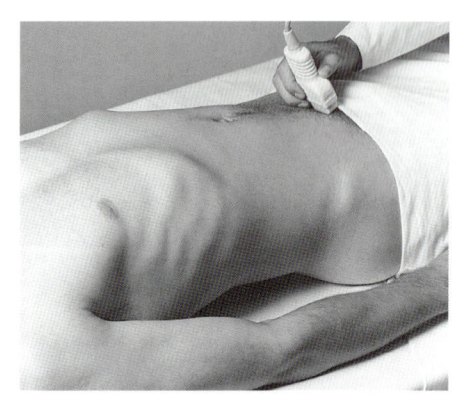

Fig. 54.2 a

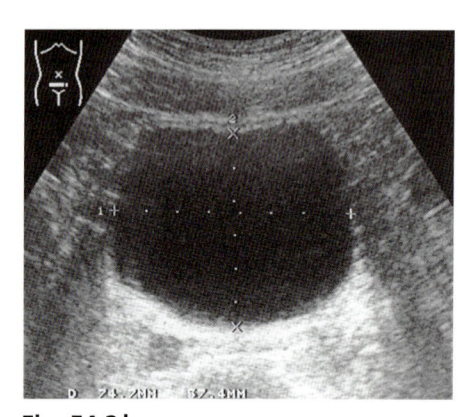

Fig. 54.2 b

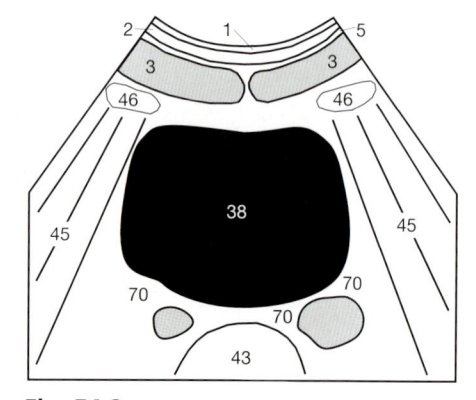

Fig. 54.2 c

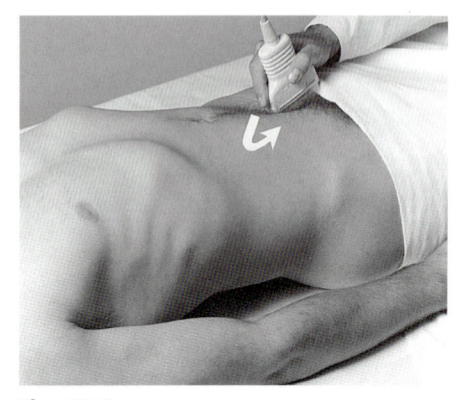

Fig. 54.3 a

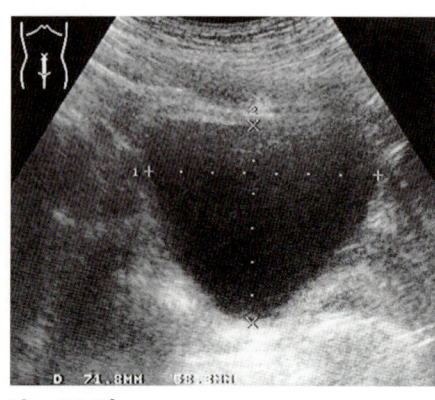

Fig. 54.3 b

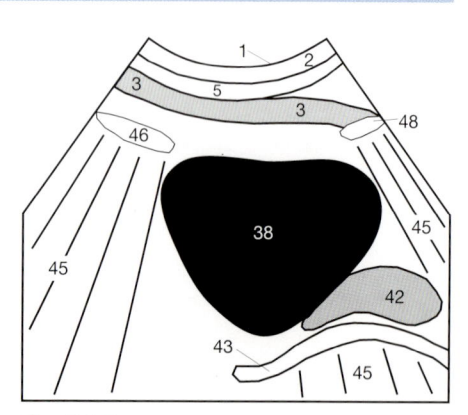

Fig. 54.3 c

8 Urinary Bladder — Indwelling Catheter, Cystitis, Sediment

The wall (77) and lumen (38) of the urinary bladder can only be adequately evaluated when the bladder is full. An indwelling catheter (76) usually results in an empty bladder (Fig. 55.1), precluding any reliable evaluation. The catheter therefore should be clamped for an extended period to achieve filling of the bladder (38). When the edema of the bladder wall (77) is rather advanced, cystitis (Fig. 55.2) can also be recognized with the bladder empty.

The wall thickness of the distended bladder should not exceed 4 mm. After voiding, the wall is irregularly thickened and measures up to 8 mm in width. Wall-based tumors or polyps can no longer be detected. Wall thickening can be caused by inflammatory edema, increased trabeculations due to prostatic hypertrophy with bladder outlet obstruction, or a space-occupying lesion.

Even the healthy bladder is never entirely echo-free. Often, reverberation artifacts (51) of the anterior abdominal wall (Fig. 55.3) are seen in the bladder (38) anteriorly, or section thickness artifacts posteriorly, simulating intraluminal matter (compare p. 10). These artifacts have to be differentiated from the real sedimentations of blood clots (52) or concrements (49) along the floor of the urinary bladder (Fig. 55.3). By rapidly changing the pressure applied to the transducer, intraluminal matter can be mechanically disturbed and made to float within the lumen. A section thickness artifact or wall-based tumor lack any response to this maneuver.

As an incidental finding, a forceful jet of urine can be propelled from the ureteral ostium into the bladder lumen. This jet phenomenon is physiologic. If transabdominal sonography is inconclusive, transrectal or vaginal transducers should be used. These endocavitary transducers generally have a better resolution because a higher frequency can be used due to the shorter distance to the target organ. These special examinations require additional expertise and training.

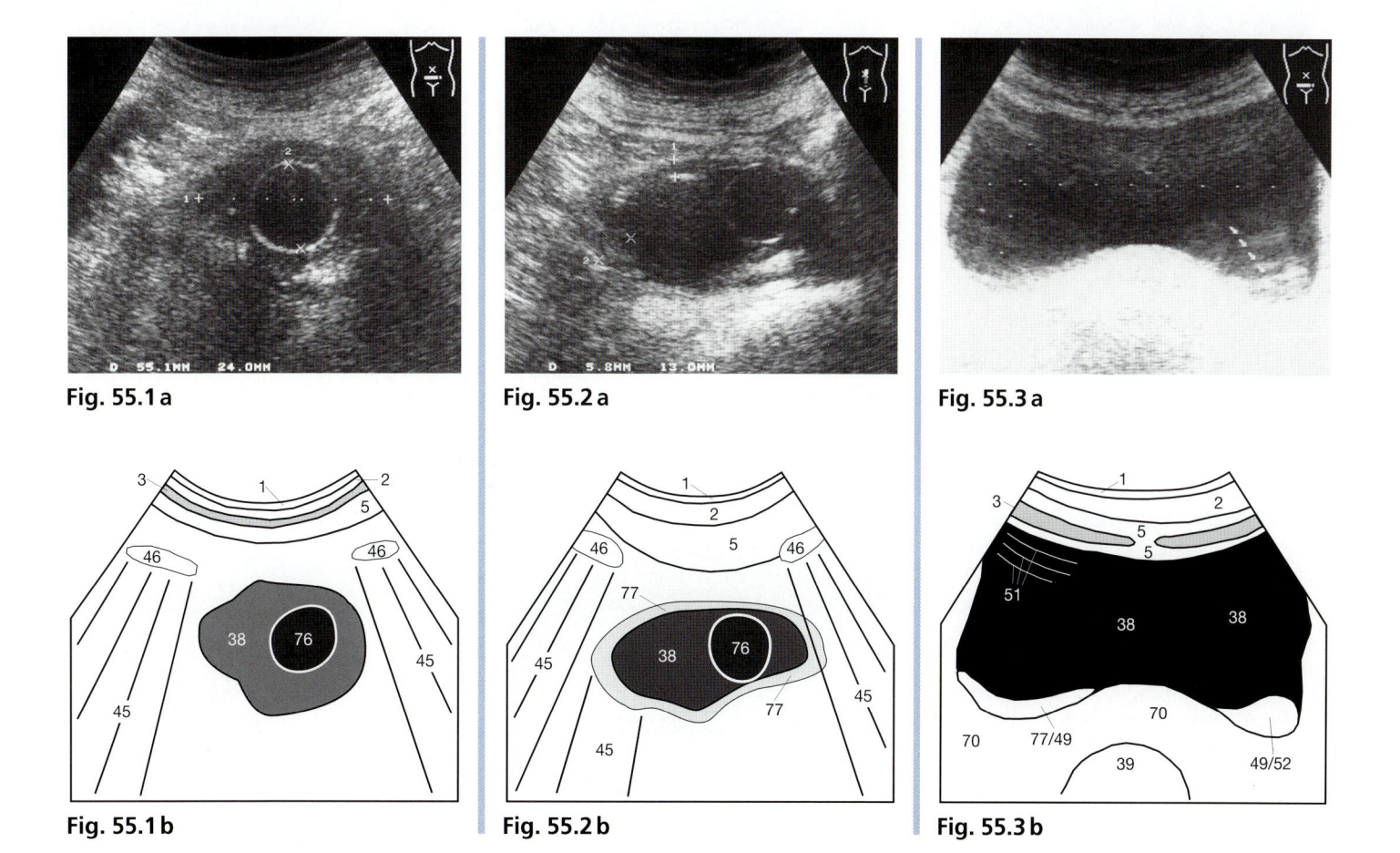

Fig. 55.1 a

Fig. 55.2 a

Fig. 55.3 a

Fig. 55.1 b

Fig. 55.2 b

Fig. 55.3 b

9 Male Genital Organs — Prostate Gland, Testicles and Scrotum

Transabdominal sonography of the genital organs requires a filled urinary bladder (38), which displaces the air-containing intestinal loops (46) cranially and laterally to avoid their interfering shadows (45) and serves as an acoustic window. The prostate gland (42) is located on the floor of the bladder anterior to the rectum (43) and is visualized on the suprapubic transverse section and on the sagittal longitudinal section (Fig. 56.1). The normal prostate gland should not exceed the approximate size of 3 x 3 x 5 cm or the approximate volume of 25 ml. In older men, an enlarged prostate gland is frequently encountered (Fig. 56.2), which interferes with voiding and can lead to a trabeculated bladder (compare Fig. 55.2).

The enlarged prostate gland (42) elevates the bladder floor (38), but the urinary bladder remains outlined by a wall that is seen as a smooth line (Fig. 56.2). Advanced prostatic hypertrophy stenoses the urethra, causing hypertrophy of the bladder wall, that beomes visible as a thick rim (77) around the bladder (Fig. 56.3). The carcinoma of the prostate gland (54) usually arises in the periphery of the gland, can infiltrate the bladder wall and extend as a lobulated mass into the lumen of the bladder (Fig. 56.3).

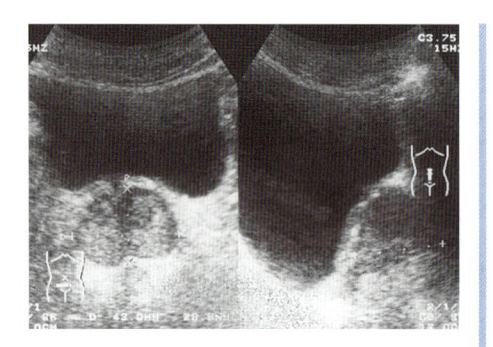

Fig. 56.1 a

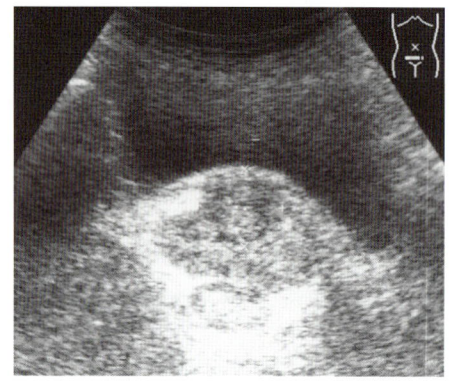

Fig. 56.2 a

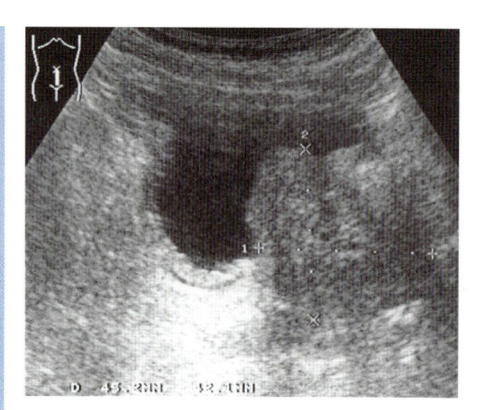

Fig. 56.3 a

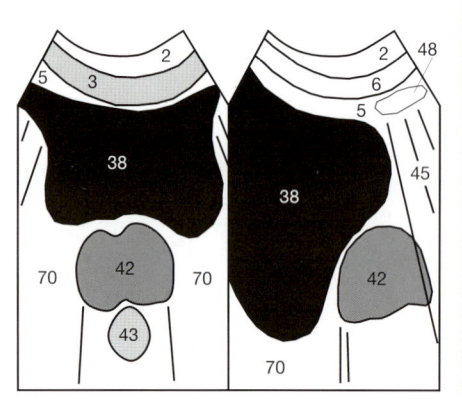

Fig. 56.1 b

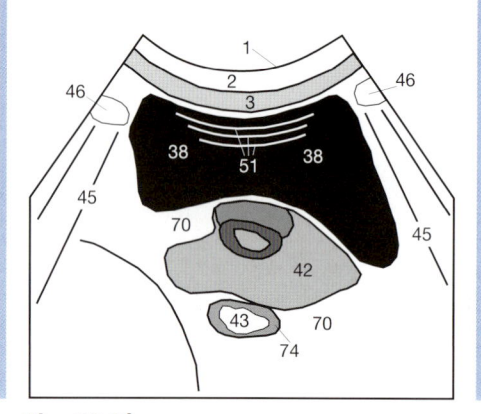

Fig. 56.2 b

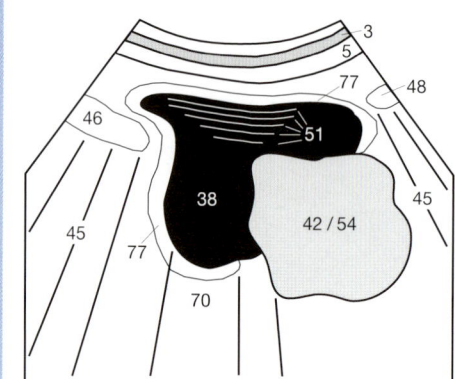

Fig. 56.3 b

The normal testicle (98) of the adult male is homogeneously hypoechoic, sharply demarcated from the layers of the scrotum (100), and measures about 3 x 4 cm (Fig. 56.4). The epididymis (99) sits on top of the upper testicular pole like a cap and extends along the posterior testicular wall. In children, both testicles should be visualized together in the scrotum on the transverse section to exclude an undescended testicle with certainty (refer to p. 57).

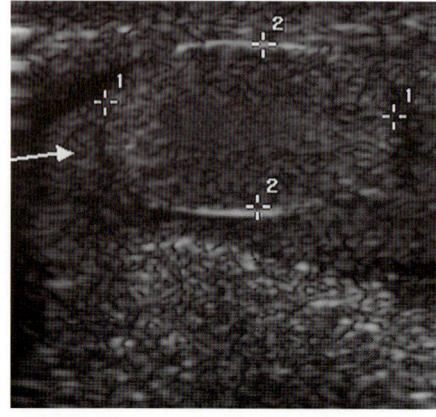

Fig. 56.4 a

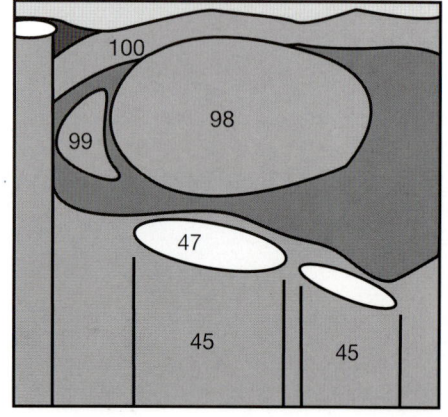

Fig. 56.4 b

9 Male Genital Organs — Undescended Testicle, Orchitis/Epididymitis

If both testicles are not found in the scrotum after the age of 3 months, the question of localizing the undescended or ectopic testicles must be addressed. Frequently, the testicle (98) is found in the inguinal canal near the anterior abdominal wall (2, 5), as seen in **Figure 57.1**. An unsuccessful sonographic detection of an undescended or ectopic testicle, which is at risk of malignant transformation, should be supplemented by an MR examination.

The sudden onset of severe scrotal pain radiating into the groin demands differential diagnostic clarification between inflammation and torsion since the ischemic tolerance of testicular tissue before irreversible necrosis is only 6 hours. In inflammation, perfusion is maintained, and can be seen by (color) Doppler sonography as a characteristic arterial flow profile (↘) in the testicular tissue **(Fig. 57.2)**, frequently increased on the affected side. Torsion, in contrast, shows decreased perfusion in relation to the other side or lacks perfusion entirely.

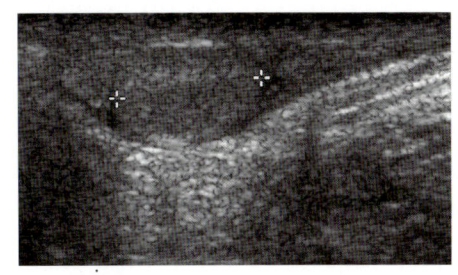

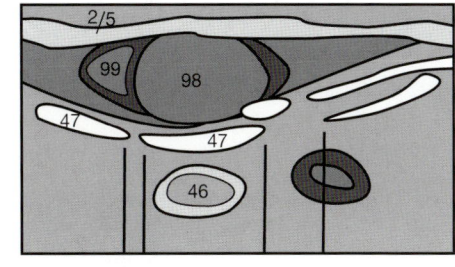

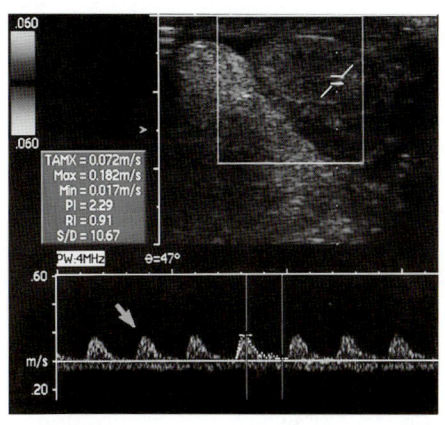

Fig. 57.1 a

Fig. 57.1 b

Fig. 57.2

Orchitis or epididymitis is usually accompanied by edematous thickening of the testicle (98) or epididymis (99) **(Fig. 57.3)**. If the findings are inconclusive, comparing both sides to determine their relative size can be helpful. A thickened and partially multilayered scrotal wall (100) can be seen as manifestation of an accompanying edematous reaction.

A homogeneous anechoic fluid collection (64) invariably represents a hydrocele **(Fig. 57.4)**. The diagnosis of a varicocele is established by the Valsalva maneuver or color-coded Doppler sonography. Occasionally, herniated bowel loops (46), a hydrocele (64), and the ipsilateral testicle (98) can be visualized together on one sonographic section **(Fig. 57.5)**. A hydrocele can accompany a testicular malignancy. Most, but not all, testicular tumors cause a heterogeneous parenchymal pattern. A well-differentiated seminoma can be homogeneous and present as an unremarkable sonographic pattern.

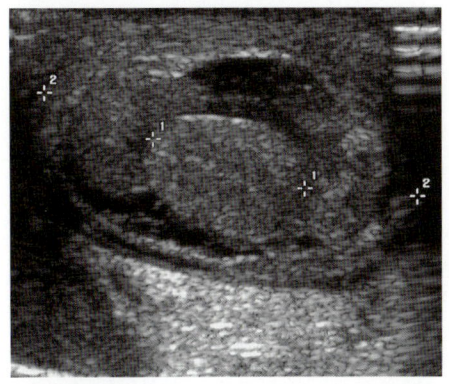

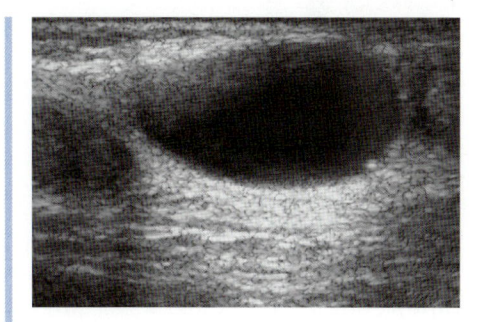

Fig. 57.3 a

Fig. 57.4 a

Fig. 57.5 a

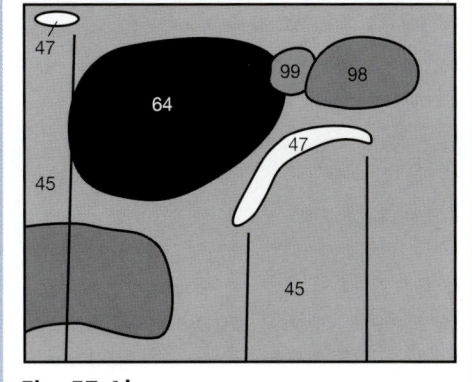

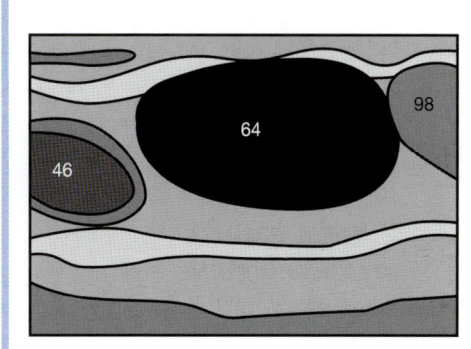

Fig. 57.3 b

Fig. 57.4 b

Fig. 57.5 b

10 Female Genital Organs

Normal Findings

To visualize the uterus (39) and ovaries (91), transabdominal sonographic imaging of the lesser pelvis requires a distended urinary bladder (38) as acoustic window (Figs. 58.1 a–c). To achieve the necessary depth penetration, low frequencies (3.5–3.75 MHz) with the corresponding decreased spatial resolution have to be selected (refer to p. 8).

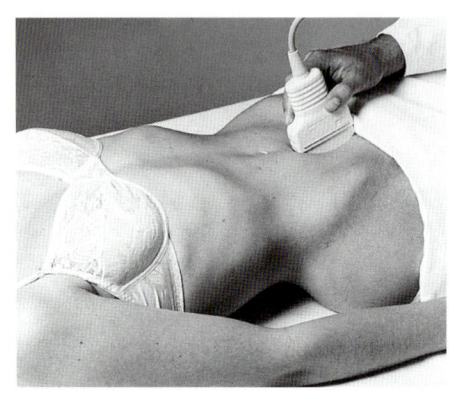

Fig. 58.1 a

Fig. 58.1 b

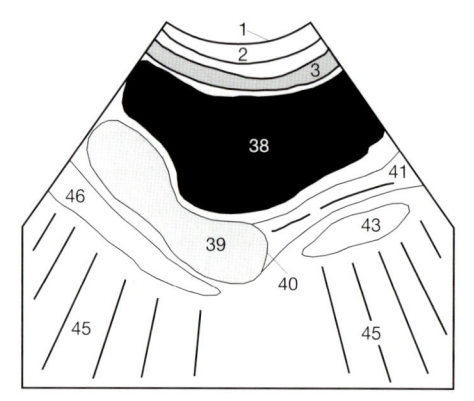

Fig. 58.1 c

Better visualization can be accomplished by using endovaginal probes (Fig. 58.2 a), which can be positioned close to the target organs of the uterus (39) and ovaries (91) (Fig. 58.3 a) and can be operated at higher frequencies (5–10 MHz) with a correspondingly higher spatial resolution. Transvaginal sonography can be performed without a filled urinary bladder.

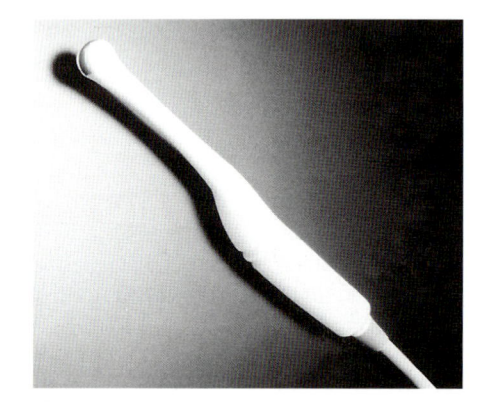

Fig. 58.2 a

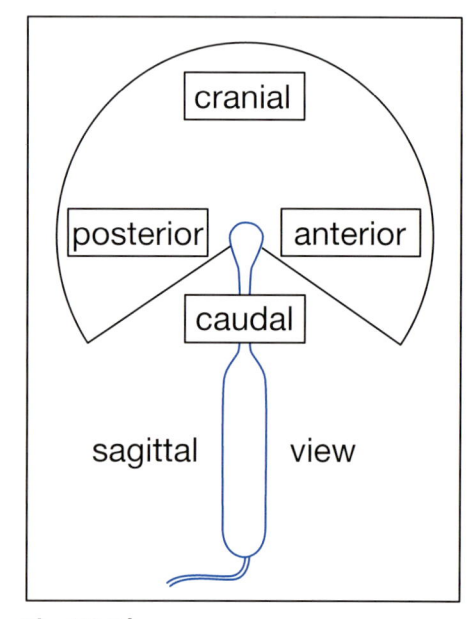

Fig. 58.2 b

In comparison to transabdominal images, the images are acquired from below and the endovaginal images are seen "upside down." The sound waves propagate from the probe (located inferiorly in the body and at the inferior border of the images) upward (superiorly). This orientation, to which the novice is unaccustomed, shows the urinary bladder (38) and the anterior abdominal wall (1–3) at the upper border on coronal images, far away from the probe. On sagittal sections (Fig. 58.3), the urinary bladder is on the right side of the image if viewed from the right side of the patient. Some examiners prefer the images as viewed from the left side, with the anterior structures then seen on the left side of the image.

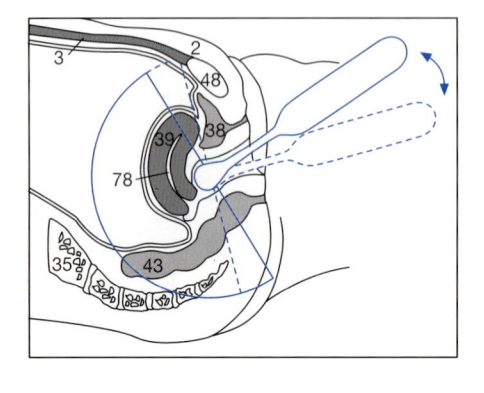

Fig. 58.3 a

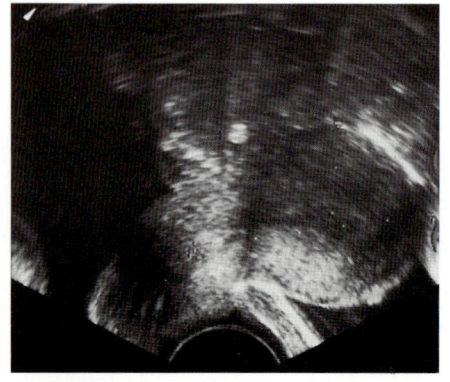

Fig. 58.3 b

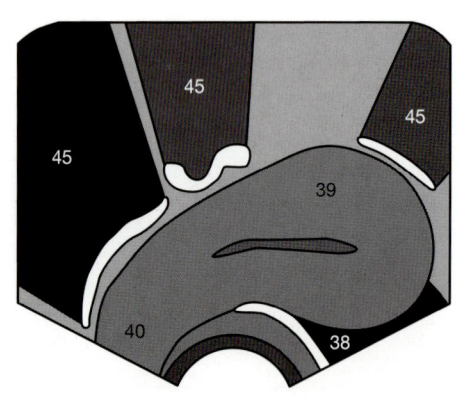

Fig. 58.3 c

10 Female Genital Organs — Uterus

The width of the endometrium (78) varies with the menstrual cycle: immediately after menstruation, a thin, echogenic, linear echo is seen **(Fig. 59.1)**. At the time of ovulation, the endometrium is separated from the myometrium (39) by an echogenic rim (∠) **(Fig. 59.2)**. After ovulation, the midline echo (→) gradually disappears in the secretory endometrium **(Fig. 59.3)** until only an echogenic endometrium is recognized.

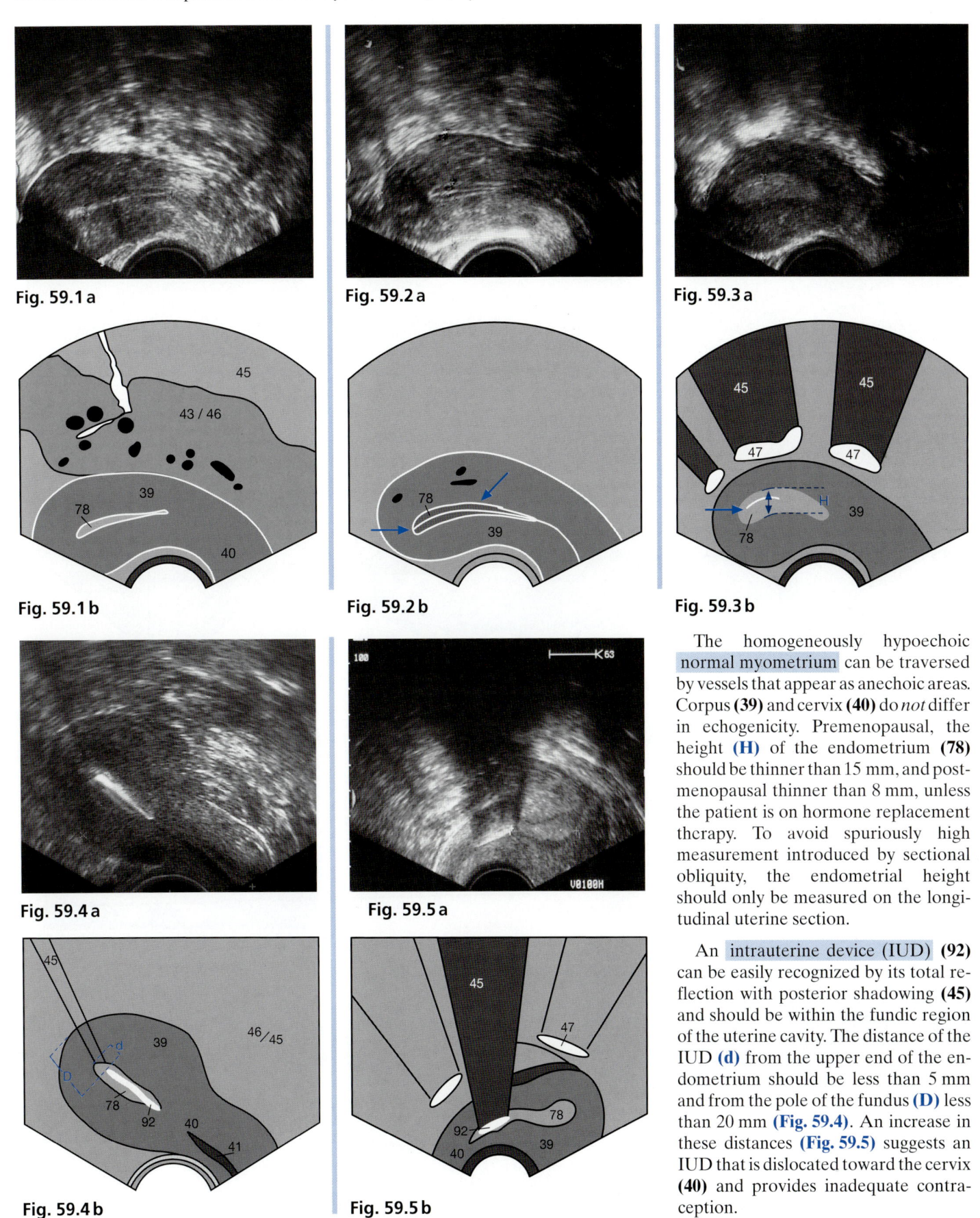

Fig. 59.1 a

Fig. 59.2 a

Fig. 59.3 a

Fig. 59.1 b

Fig. 59.2 b

Fig. 59.3 b

The homogeneously hypoechoic normal myometrium can be traversed by vessels that appear as anechoic areas. Corpus (39) and cervix (40) do *not* differ in echogenicity. Premenopausal, the height **(H)** of the endometrium (78) should be thinner than 15 mm, and postmenopausal thinner than 8 mm, unless the patient is on hormone replacement therapy. To avoid spuriously high measurement introduced by sectional obliquity, the endometrial height should only be measured on the longitudinal uterine section.

Fig. 59.4 a

Fig. 59.5 a

An intrauterine device (IUD) (92) can be easily recognized by its total reflection with posterior shadowing (45) and should be within the fundic region of the uterine cavity. The distance of the IUD **(d)** from the upper end of the endometrium should be less than 5 mm and from the pole of the fundus **(D)** less than 20 mm **(Fig. 59.4)**. An increase in these distances **(Fig. 59.5)** suggests an IUD that is dislocated toward the cervix (40) and provides inadequate contraception.

Fig. 59.4 b

Fig. 59.5 b

10 Female Genital Organs — Tumors of the Uterus

The normal uterus is demarcated by an echogenic serosa and exhibits a homogeneously hypoechoic myometrium (39). The most common benign uterine tumors, the fibroids (myomas), arise from the smooth musculature and are usually located in the corpus of the uterus. For planning the surgical enucleation of fibroids, it is relevant to distinguish intra-/transmural (Fig. 60.1) and submucosal (Fig. 60.2) fibroids from subserosal fibroids on the surface of the uterus (Fig. 60.3) (54). The submucosal location close to the uterine cavity can easily mistaken for endometrial polyps (65). Fibroids usually have a homogeneous or a concentrically lamellated echo pattern with distinct demarcation and a smooth surface, but can contain calcifications with corresponding acoustic shadowing or a central necrosis. The size of fibroids should always be measured and controlled by serial examinations to discover the rare sarcomatous transformation by revealing any rapid growth. Only in early pregnancy can a sudden increase in size be attributed to a benign lesion.

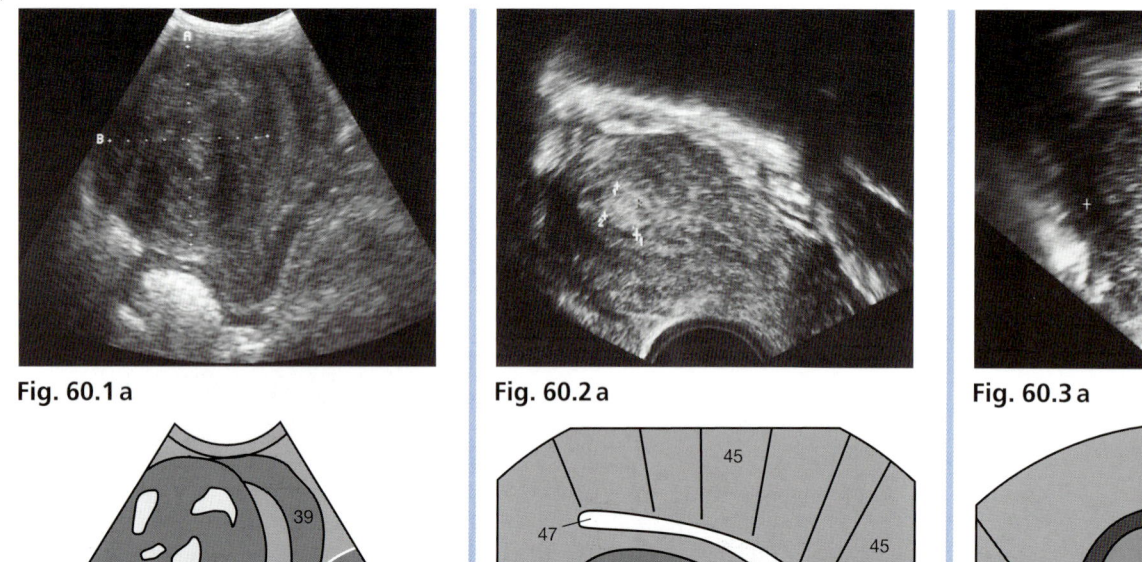

Fig. 60.1 a

Fig. 60.2 a

Fig. 60.3 a

Fig. 60.1 b

Fig. 60.2 b

Fig. 60.3 b

In menopause, hormone replacement therapy with estrogen can lead to estrogen producing ovarian tumors, or persistent follicles can induce endometrial hyperplasia (Fig. 60.4), which can eventually transform adenocarcinoma (54) if the high estrogen levels are maintained (Fig. 60.6). Malignant criteria include conspicuous endometrial thickness exceeding 15 or 8 mm (premenopausal and postmenopausal, respectively), a heterogeneous echogenicity, and an irregular outline (Fig. 60.6). A hypoechoic collection of blood (✓) in the uterine cavity (hematometra, Fig. 60.5) can be caused both by postinflammatory adhesions at the cervical os, for instance after conization, and by a cervix tumor.

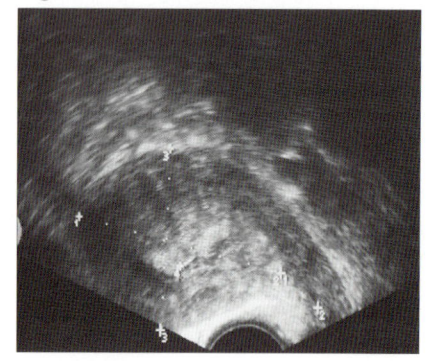

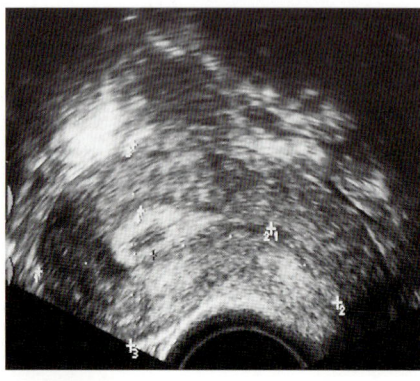

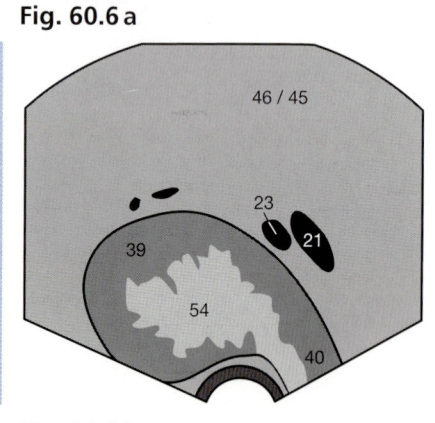

Fig. 60.6 a

Fig. 60.4

Fig. 60.5

Fig. 60.6 b

10 Female Genital Organs — Ovaries

The ovaries (91) are visualized on craniolaterally oriented sagittal sections and are frequently in the immediate vicinity of the iliac vessels (23) as seen in **Figure 61.1**. To measure the volume of the ovaries, a transverse section has to be added. The three diameters multiplied by 0.5 approximate the ovarian volume: in the adult female these volumes are between 5.5 and 10.0 cm³ for each ovary, with a mean value of just less than 8 cm³. The ovarian volume does not change during pregnancy, but decreases steadily by about 3.5 to 2.5 cm³ postmenopausally, relating to the length of time after the menopause.

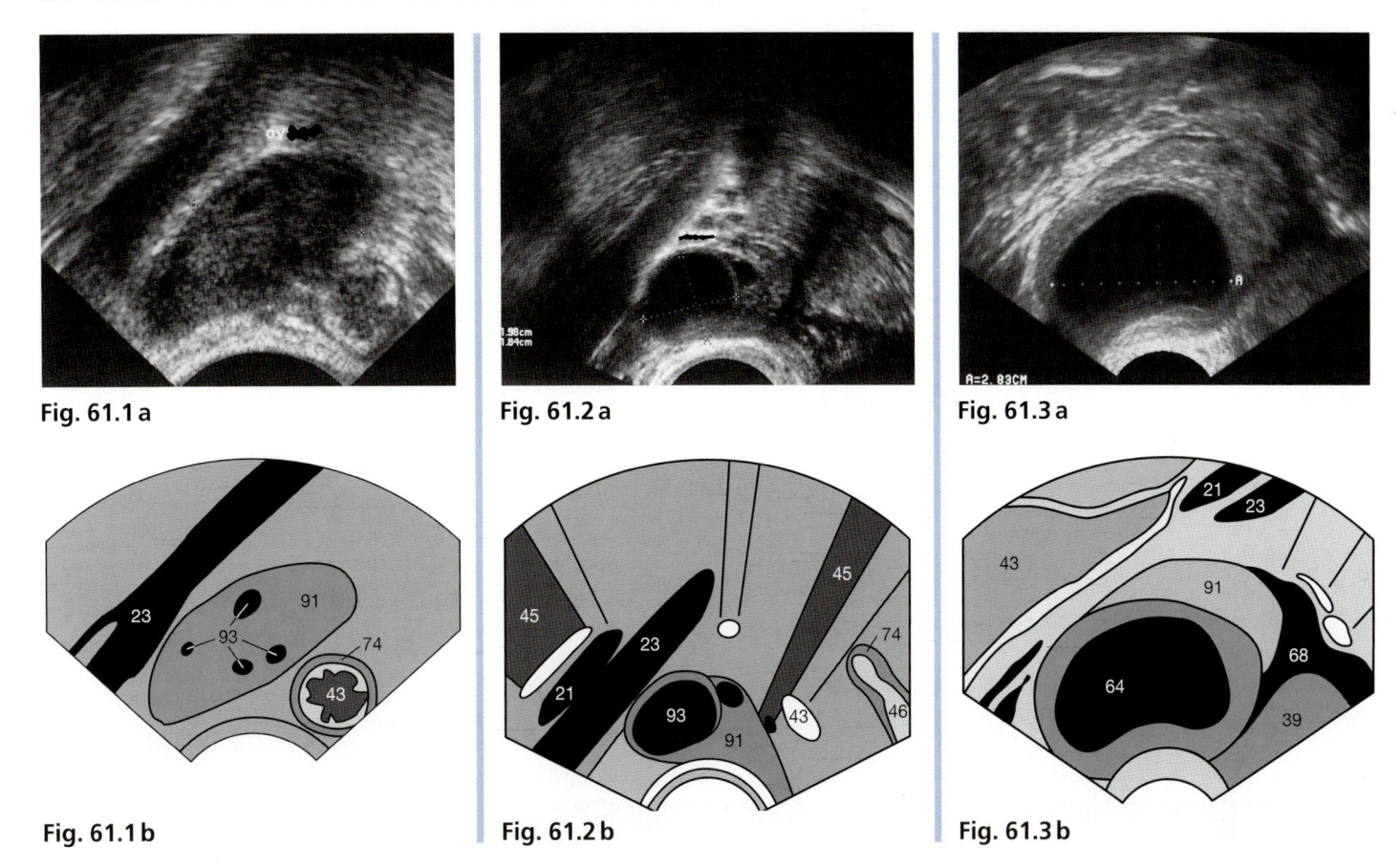

Fig. 61.1 a

Fig. 61.2 a

Fig. 61.3 a

Fig. 61.1 b

Fig. 61.2 b

Fig. 61.3 b

Normally, several follicles (93) are detectable in the 1st days of the menstrual cycle, seen as 4–6-mm small cycsts in the ovary. After the 10th day of the cycle, one follicle becomes dominant, the so-called graafian follicle, with a diameter of about 10 mm **(Fig. 61.2)**. Thereafter, this follicle shows linear growth, increasing in size by about 2 mm per day until it reaches a size of 18–25 mm just before ovulation. In the meantime the other follicles regress.

It is relevant for fertility therapy and IVF that serial sonographic examinations allow close monitoring of follicular maturation, and that the time of the ovulation might be observed by endovaginal sonography. Signs considered to indicate imminent ovulation include a follicular size exceeding 2 cm, the visualization of the small, peripheral, ring-shaped cumulus oophorus, and intrafollicular echos projecting from the wall. Following ovulation, the leading graafian follicle "disappears" or at least diminishes markedly in size; at the same time a small amount of free fluid can be detected in the cul-de-sac. Through invasion of capillary sprouts, the ruptured follicle becomes the progesterone-producing corpus luteum, which remains visible for only a few days as a hyperechoic area at the site of the former graafian follicle. In case of fertilization and implantation, the corpus luteum persists and can be identified as a corpus luteum cyst (64) until the 14th gestational week **(Fig. 61.3)**.

Follicular dysfunction includes premature luteinization of the follicle and continued growth without ovulation to a follicle cyst (64) **(Fig. 61.4)**. The diagnosis of a follicle cyst should be considered if the diameter is larger than 3 cm.

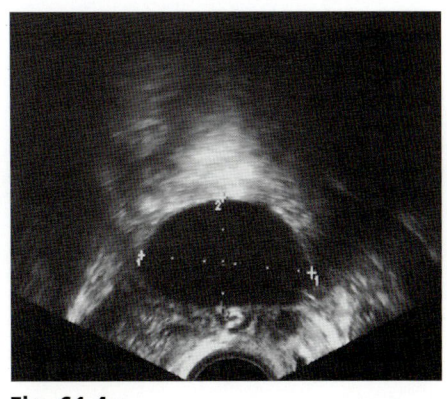

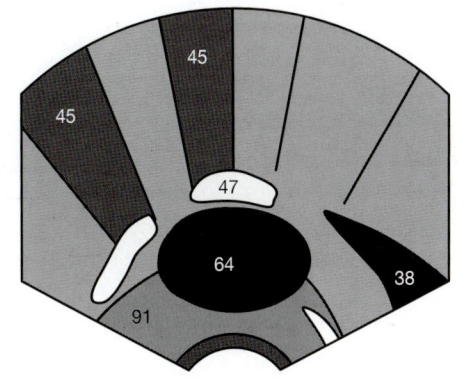

Fig. 61.4 a

Fig. 61.4 b

10 Female Genital Organs — Ovaries

An ovarian cyst with a diameter exceeding 5 cm is suspicious of tumorous growth and, especially if septations, wall thickening, or solid internal echos (↖) are present **(64)** **(Fig. 62.1)**, malignancy must be ruled out. A cyst containing sebum, hair, or other tissue components (↘) constitutes a dermoid **(Fig. 62.2)**, which comprises about 15% of the usually unilateral ovarian tumors and can be classified as a primary benign tumor that rarely undergoes malignant transformation. A dermoid has to be distinguished from hemorrhagic or endometrial cysts, which are filled with blood products and can exhibit fluid–fluid interfaces (→) **(Fig. 62.3)** or a homogeneous echo pattern **(50)** **(Fig. 62.4)**.

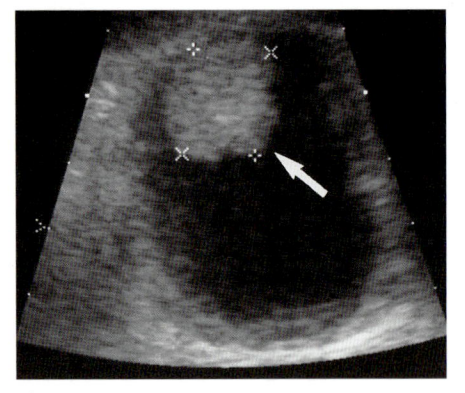

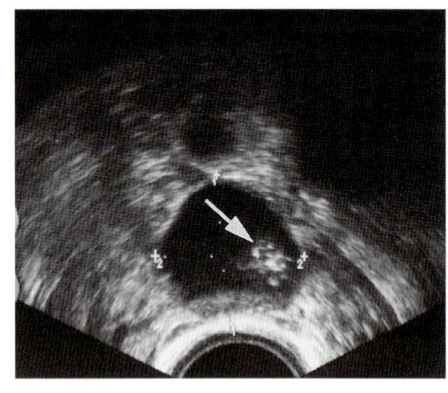

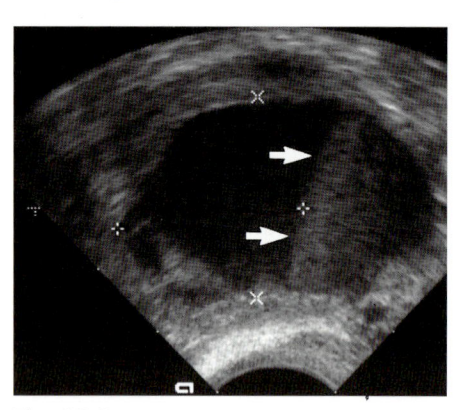

Fig. 62.1

Fig. 62.2

Fig. 62.3

In a cycle stimulated as part of infertility therapy, merely measuring the serum hormone levels can neither rule out hyperstimulated ovaries **(Fig. 62.5)** nor reliably estimate the number of preovulatory follicles **(93)**. It is for this reason that the number of maturing graafian follicles be monitored sonographically so that therapy can be terminated and contraceptive measures advised when more than two preovulatory follicles develop.

About 5% of women have polycystic ovarian syndrome (PCOS) caused by inhibited follicular maturation. Its most common cause is adrenal androgen excess. It is characteristic of PCOS for the ovary **(91)** to contain several small cysts **(64)**, predominantly around the periphery where they form a "pearls on a string" appearance within tissue of increased echogenicity **(Fig. 62.6)**.

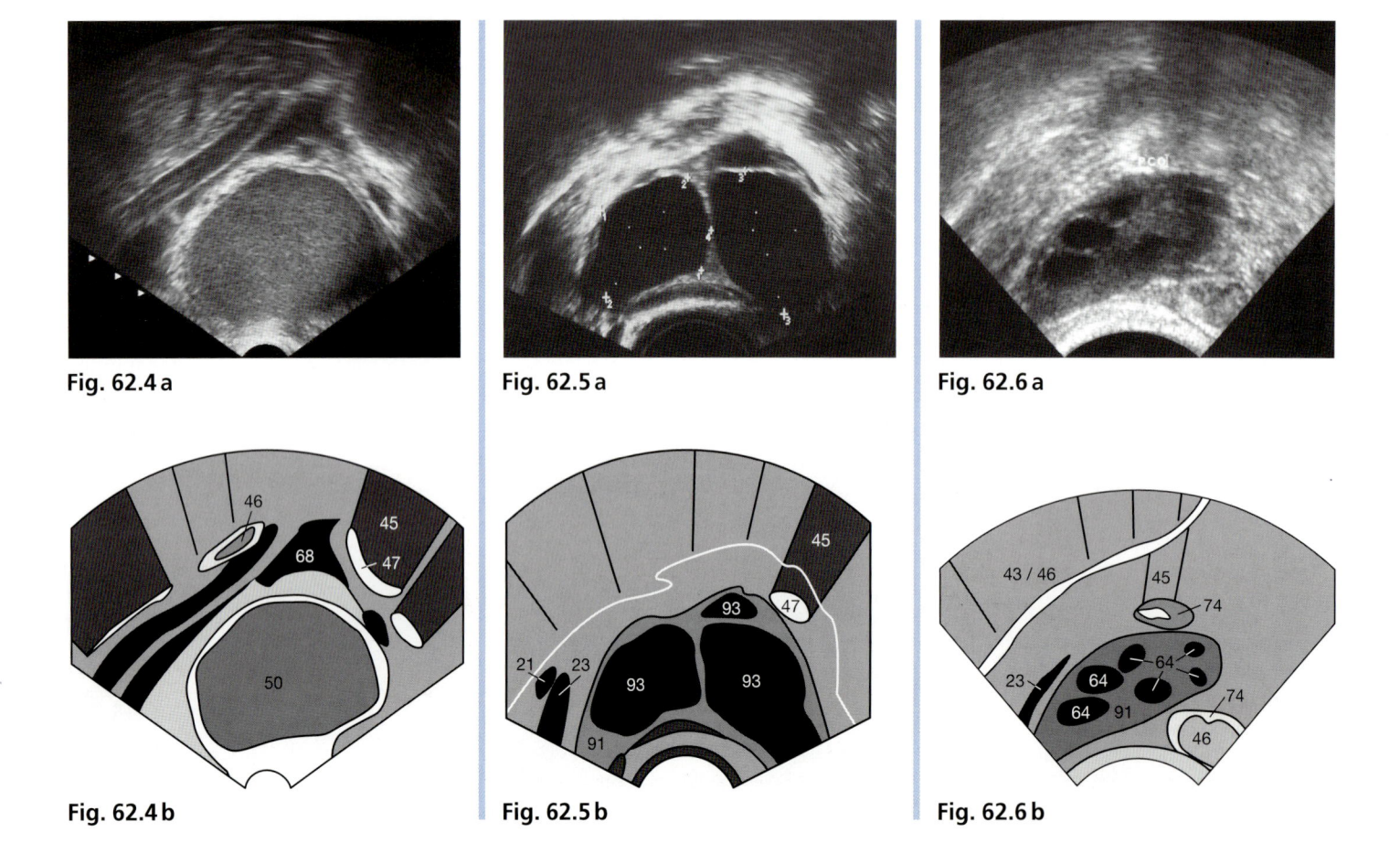

Fig. 62.4 a

Fig. 62.5 a

Fig. 62.6 a

Fig. 62.4 b

Fig. 62.5 b

Fig. 62.6 b

11 Pregnancy

Diagnosis of Early Pregnancy

An elevated β-HCG in the maternal serum or urine is an indication of pregnancy, and sonography can confirm the pregnancy. Furthermore, sonography can identify multiple pregnancy (refer to Figs. 66.3, 66.4), which is not always hormonally recognized, and it can exclude ectopic pregnancy (EP).

Vaginal sonography can detect early intrauterine pregnancy (Fig. 63.1) when the gestational sac (chorionic cavity) measures 2 to 3 mm in diameter. This size is generally found at the beginning of the 4th gestational week plus 3 days after the last menstrual period or 14 days after conception. The initially small cavity grows at a rate of about 1.1 mm per day to become the amniotic cavity (101), in which the embryo (95) is later detectable (Fig. 63.2).

A gestational sac (chorionic cavity) (101) outside the uterus (39) constitutes an ectopic pregnancy (Fig. 63.3).

Fetal cardiac activity can be detected from the 6th gestational week. At this time, the normal rate is about 80 to 90 beats per minute.

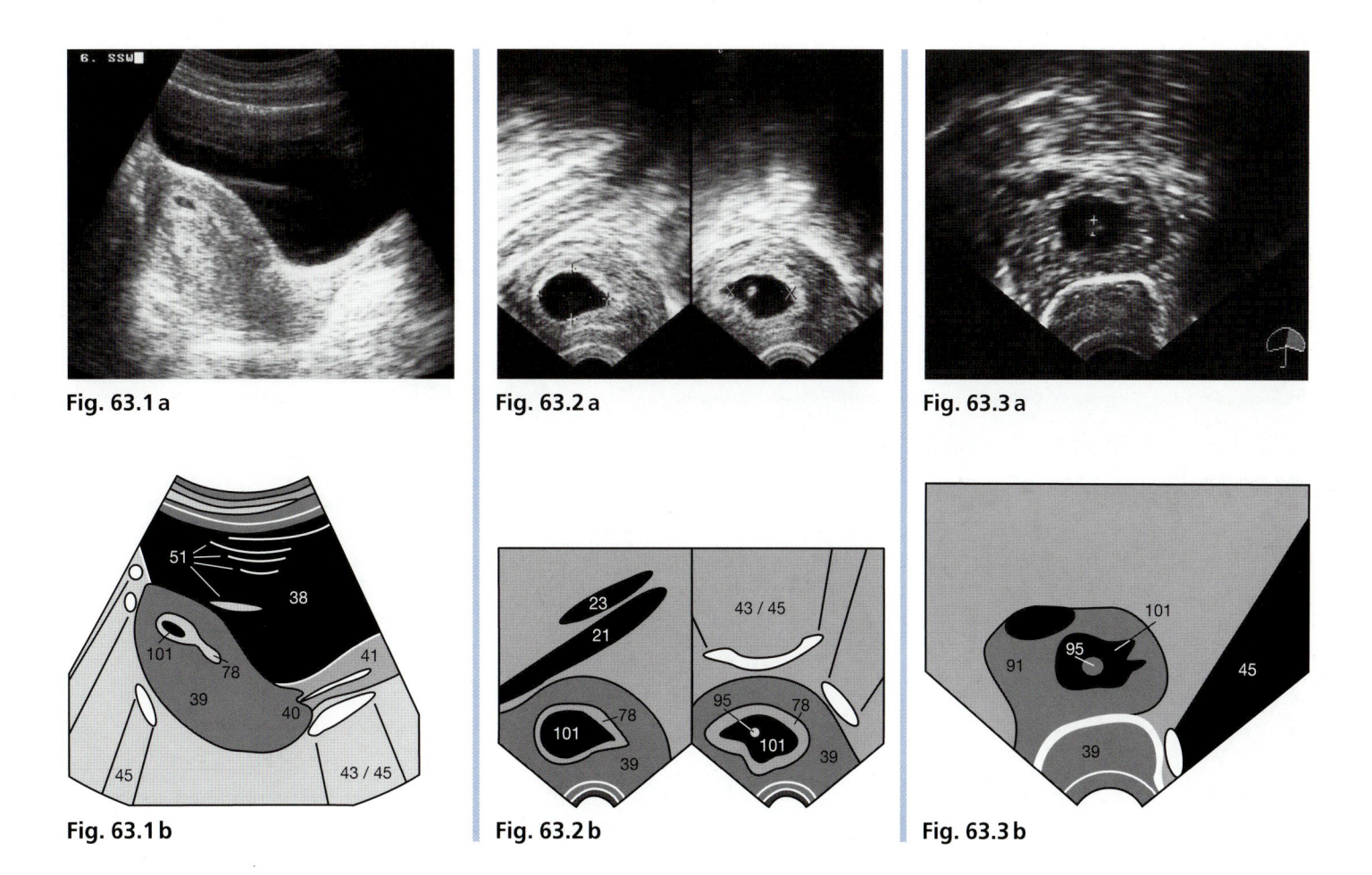

Fig. 63.1 a

Fig. 63.2 a

Fig. 63.3 a

Fig. 63.1 b

Fig. 63.2 b

Fig. 63.3 b

Biophysical limits: According to the guidelines of the American Institute of Ultrasound in Medicine (AIUM), acoustic energies below 100 mW/cm² or less than 50 J/cm have no confirmed biologic effect and can be considered safe [1]. Since the sonographic exposure delivered with conventional real time sonography is far below those values, neither thermal nor cavitation effects are to be expected.

The bioeffects are different for color-coded Doppler sonography and PW (pulsed-wave) Doppler sonography: long examination times approach or even exceed the recommended tissue exposure limits. Though no adverse biologic effects have been reported so far with these higher sonographic tissue exposures, it is prudent to refrain from nonessential (color-) Doppler sonography during the sensitive phase of organogenesis (1st trimester) [2, 3].

1 AIUM Bioeffects Committee: Bioeffects considerations for safety in ultrasound. J Ultrasound Med., Suppl. 7 (1988): 1–38
2 Watchdog-Tutorial: Gepulste Doppler-Geräte—Sicherheitsaspekte. Ultraschall Klin. Prax. 7 (1992): 86–87
3 European Committee for Ultrasound Radiation Safety—the Watchdogs. Transvaginal ultrasonography—safety aspects. Europ J Ultrasound 1 (1994): 355–357

11 Pregnancy

Biometry In the First Trimester

In the sonographic evaluation of pregnancy, biometry is primarily used to asses intrauterine growth retardation but also assists in diagnosing anomalies. The normal biometric values for the gestational age and their percentiles are also found as tables at the end of the book.

Gestational sac (chorionic cavity) diameter (GSD): The initially anechoic chorionic cavity (101) becomes surrounded by an echogenic rim of reactic endometrium (78) (Fig. 64.1) and is detectable after the 14th day of conception. It should be detectable if the serum HCG exceeds about 750–1000 U/l—otherwise an ectopic pregnancy must be excluded (compare p. 63).

The yolk sac is seen as echoic ring–like structure at about the 5th gestational week and increases to 5 mm in size by the 10th gestational week. A diameter of the yolk sac of less than 3 mm or more than 7 mm is associated with a higher risk of developmental anomalies. A yolk sac clearly seen within the uterine cavity excludes an ectopic pregnancy since the yolk sac is fetal in origin. Figure 64.2 shows a yolk sac (102) adjacent to the spine (35) in a fetus of a gestational age of 7 weeks and 6 days.

Crown-rump length (CRL): A normal fetus is detectable at a gestational age of 6 weeks and 3 days, and has a CRL of approximately 5 mm. At this time, the amniotic cavity measures 15–18 mm. As soon as the fetus (95) is visible, the CRL replaces the GSD since it more accurately determines the gestational age (within the range of a few days) up to the 12th gestational week (Fig. 64.3). Thereafter, measuring the biparietal diameter of the head (BPD) becomes more accurate (compare p. 65).

If a fetus is not detectable in the chorionic cavity as expected for gestational age, the calculation of gestational age should be checked first. If follow-up examination fails to show appropriate development of the still empty chorionic cavity, the finding may indicate a blighted ovum without a developing fetus, which occurs with an incidence of about 5% of all gestations.

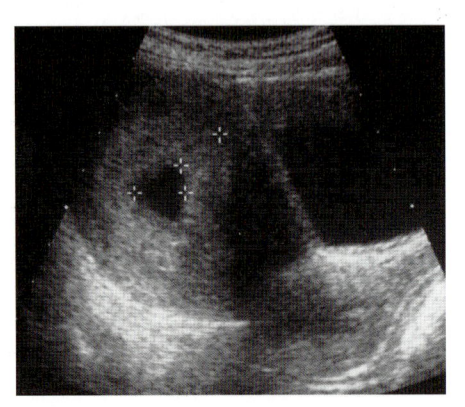

Fig. 64.1 a

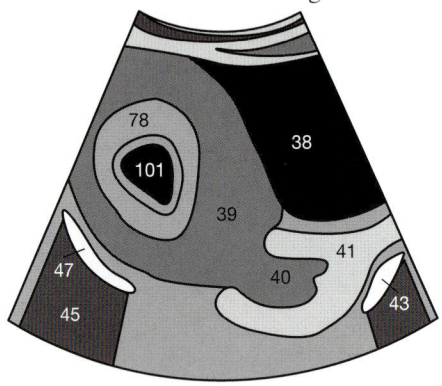

Fig. 64.1 b

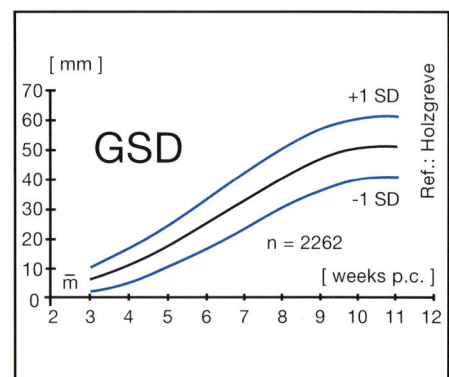

Fig. 64.1 c

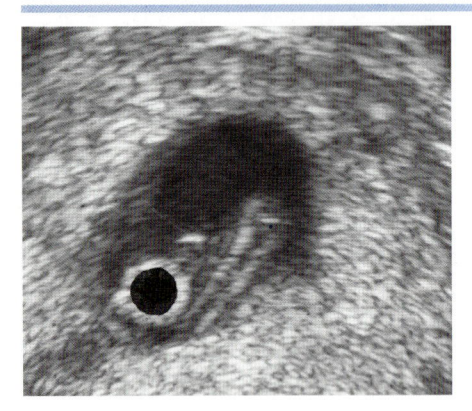

Fig. 64.2 a

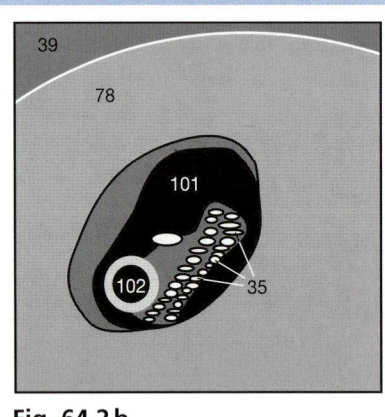

Fig. 64.2 b

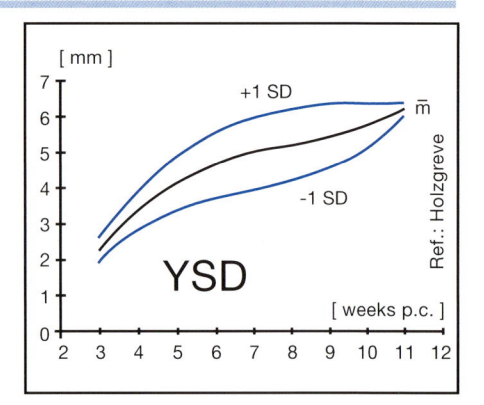

Fig. 64.2 c

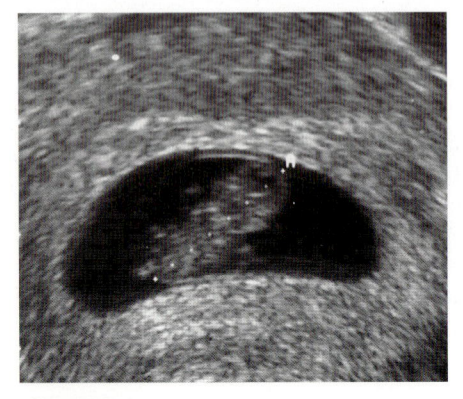

Fig. 64.3 a

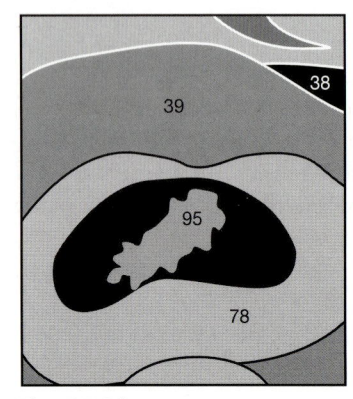

Fig. 64.3 b

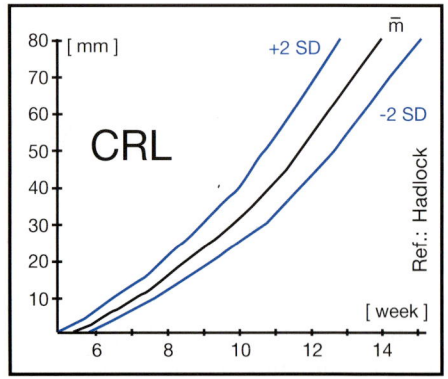

Fig. 64.3 c

11 Pregnancy — Biomety In the Second and Third Trimester

Biparietal diameter (BPD): Beginning with the 12th gestational week, measuring the BPD becomes feasible and more accurate than measuring the CRL. At this time, the choroid plexus **(104)** appears bilaterally and is seen as an echogenic structure. To make the measurement reproducible and accurate, the same reference plane **(Fig. 65.1)** should be selected, with visualization of the entire circumference of the oval skull **(105)**. It is important to select an orientation parallel to the midline echo of the falx **(106)**, which is interrupted in the anterior third by the cavum septi pellucidi. Cerebellum or orbits should *not* be in the imaging plane because the diameter would be measured too far inferiorly. In the same imaging plane, the occipitofrontal diameter (OFD) and the head circumference (HC) can be measured as well. The respective normal values can be found at the end of the book.

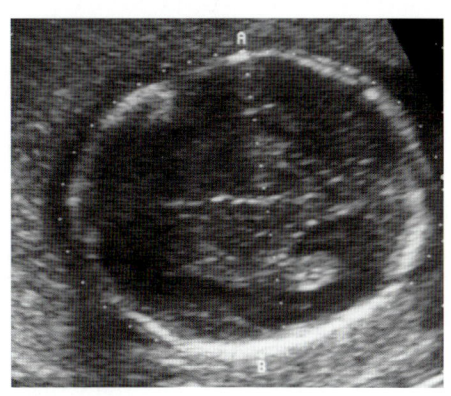

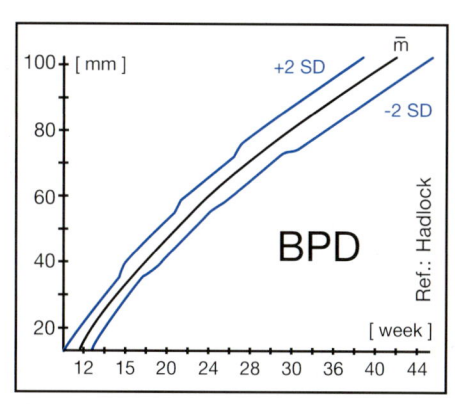

Fig. 65.1 a

Fig. 65.1 b

Fig. 65.1 c

Femoral length (FL): The ossified femoral diaphysis **(107)** is easily measured: The upper leg **(108)** should be as close as possible to the probe and oriented lengthwise, thus perpendicular to the axis of the probe **(Fig. 65.2)**. Measuring the length of the remaining tubular bones to exclude growth retardation or malformation is only necessary if the FL falls outside the reference range or if the percentile changes on sequential examinations.

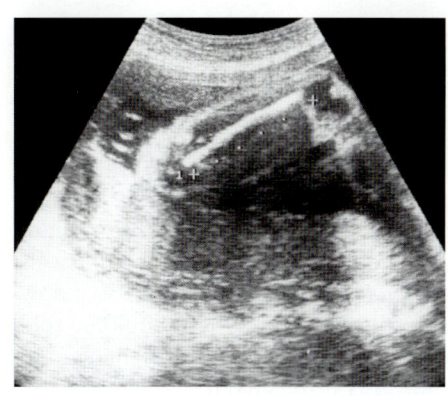

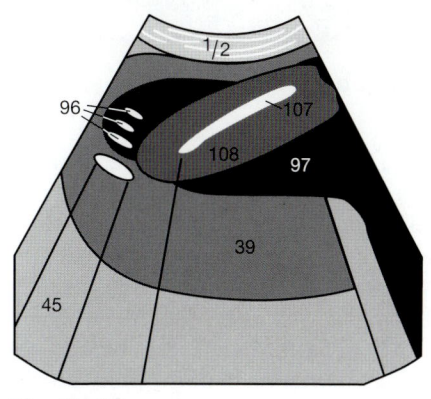

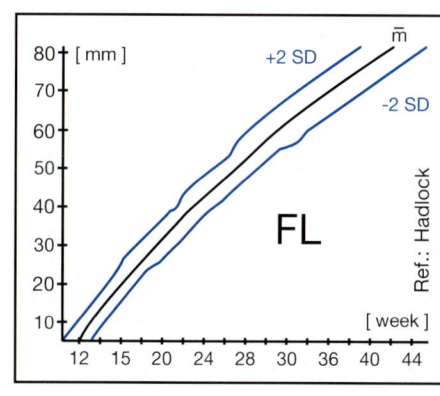

Fig. 65.2 a

Fig. 65.2 b

Fig. 65.2 c

Abdominal circumference (AC): The reference plane **(Fig. 65.3)** is the level of the liver **(9)**, possibly with visualization of the dorsal third of the umbilical and portal veins **(11)**. The bilateral ribs should be displayed symmetrically to assure that the section was not obtained in an oblique plane.

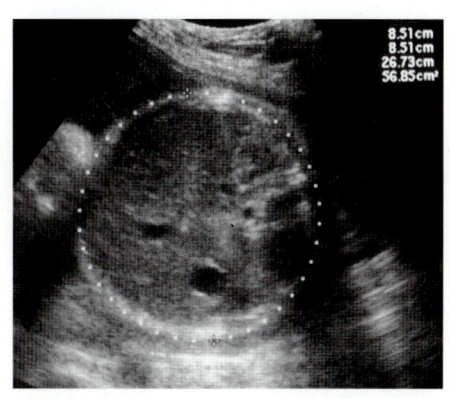

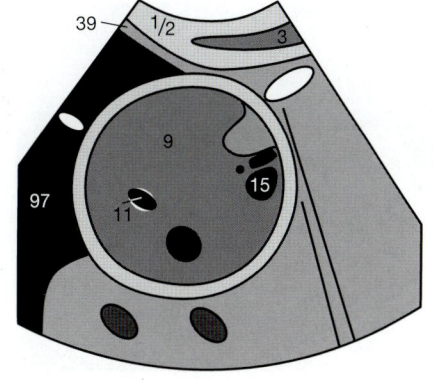

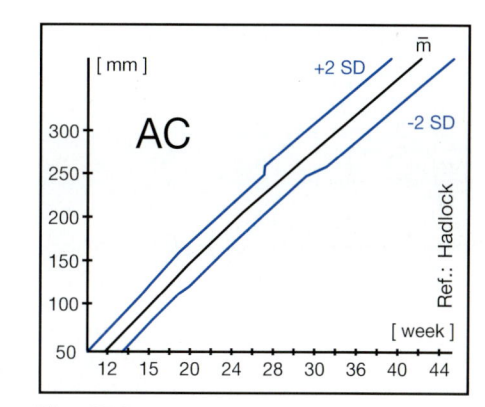

Fig. 65.3 a

Fig. 65.3 b

Fig. 65.3 c

11 Pregnancy

Placental Location and Fetal Gender

The normal location of the placenta is near the fundus of the uterus along the anterior or posterior wall. In about 20% of cases one or several unicameral cysts or cyst–like spaces **(64)** appear within the placenta **(94)** **(Fig. 66.1)** and generally are inconsequential, though a certain association with maternal diabetes or rhesus incompatibility has been proposed. The placental location should not be definitively assessed before the end of the 2nd trimester since the placenta previa of an early pregnancy can become a normal or "low" lying placenta due to stretching of the uterine cervix (distance to the internal cervical os < 5 cm).

Depending on its relationship to the cervix **(40)**, the placenta previa can be classified into three categories: total placenta previa, which covers the entire internal cervical os; partial placenta previa **(Fig. 66.2)**, which covers a portion of the os; and marginal placenta previa, which extends near the os. Evaluating the placental structure has become less important since the introduction of Doppler sonography, which has improved the assessment of placental and fetal perfusion.

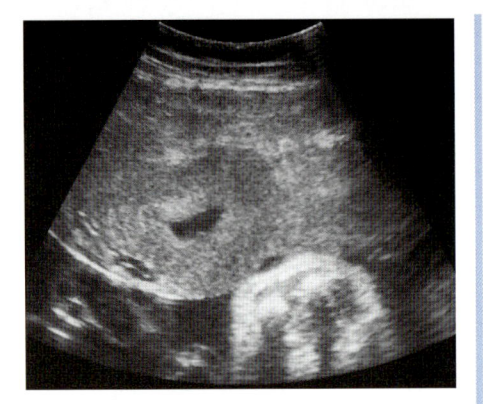

Fig. 66.1 a

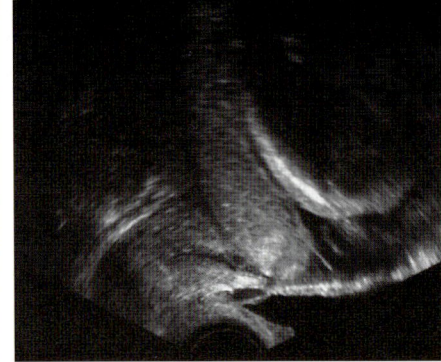

Fig. 66.2 a

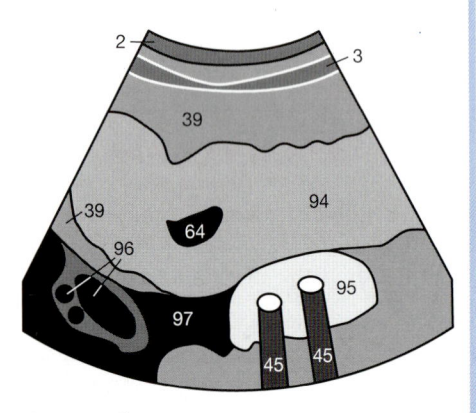

Fig. 66.1 b

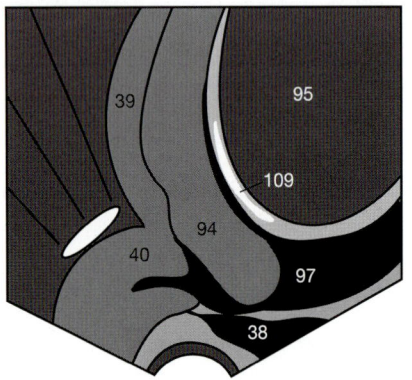

Fig. 66.2 b

In a multiple pregnancy, the placentation of the multiple gestations should be determined. The gestations **(95)** can have a common placenta (←) **(Fig. 66.4)** or their own placenta. Furthermore, the expectant parents (and their obstetrician) should be informed of a multiple pregnancy to make preparations for twins **(Fig. 66.3)** or, as the case may be, triplets **(Fig. 66.4)**. If parents wish to know whether they expect a daughter **(Fig. 66.5)** or a son **(Fig. 66.6)**, they should be told so, but only if the gender can be unequivocally determined. In early pregnancy, the umbilical cord or a hypertrophic clitoris (↘) can easily be mistaken for the penis (↖), or the female labia for the scrotum (→) **(Figs. 66.5, 66.6)**. The parents should only be told of the gender if they indicate that they wish to know.

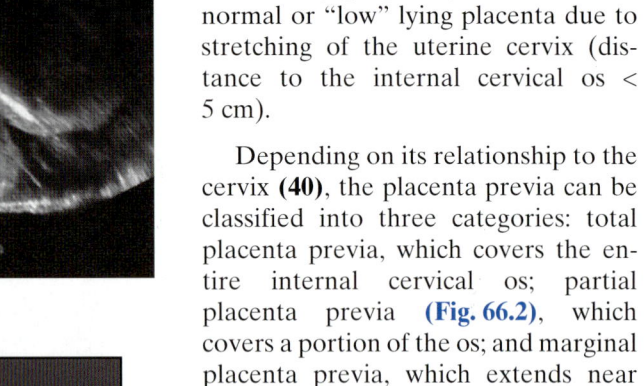

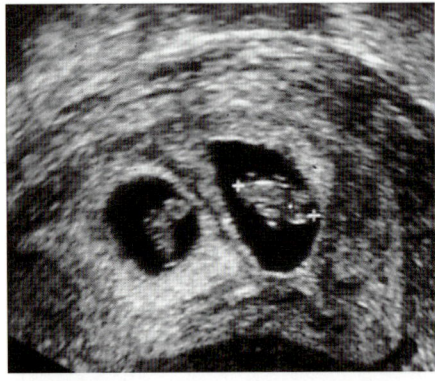

Fig. 66.3

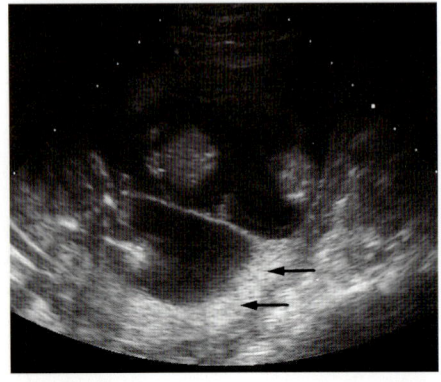

Fig. 66.4

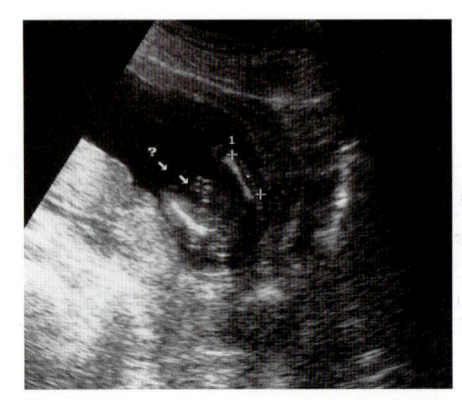

Fig. 66.5

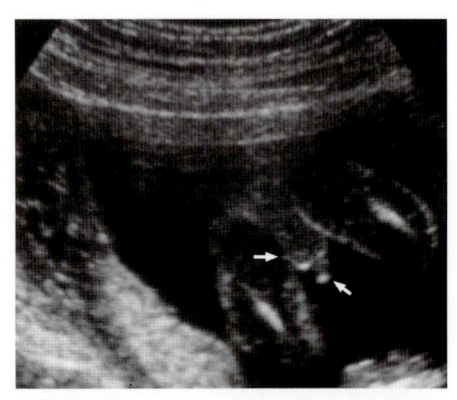

Fig. 66.6

11 Pregnancy — Diagnosis of Fetal Malformations

The cerebellum (110) is visualized on the transverse section through the posterior cerebral fossa (Fig. 67.1). A dorsal indentation (↩) should be identified. Its absence causes the cerebellum to look like a banana ("banana sign") and indicates cerebellar displacement toward the spinal canal (Fig. 67.2), suggesting a neural tube defect. For the same reason, the calvaria (105) loses its oval form on transverse sections through the cerebrum and resembles a sliced lemon ("lemon sign") with projections (✓) of the parietal bone bilaterally (Fig. 67.3). Incidentally visualized is the hyperechoic choroid plexus (104).

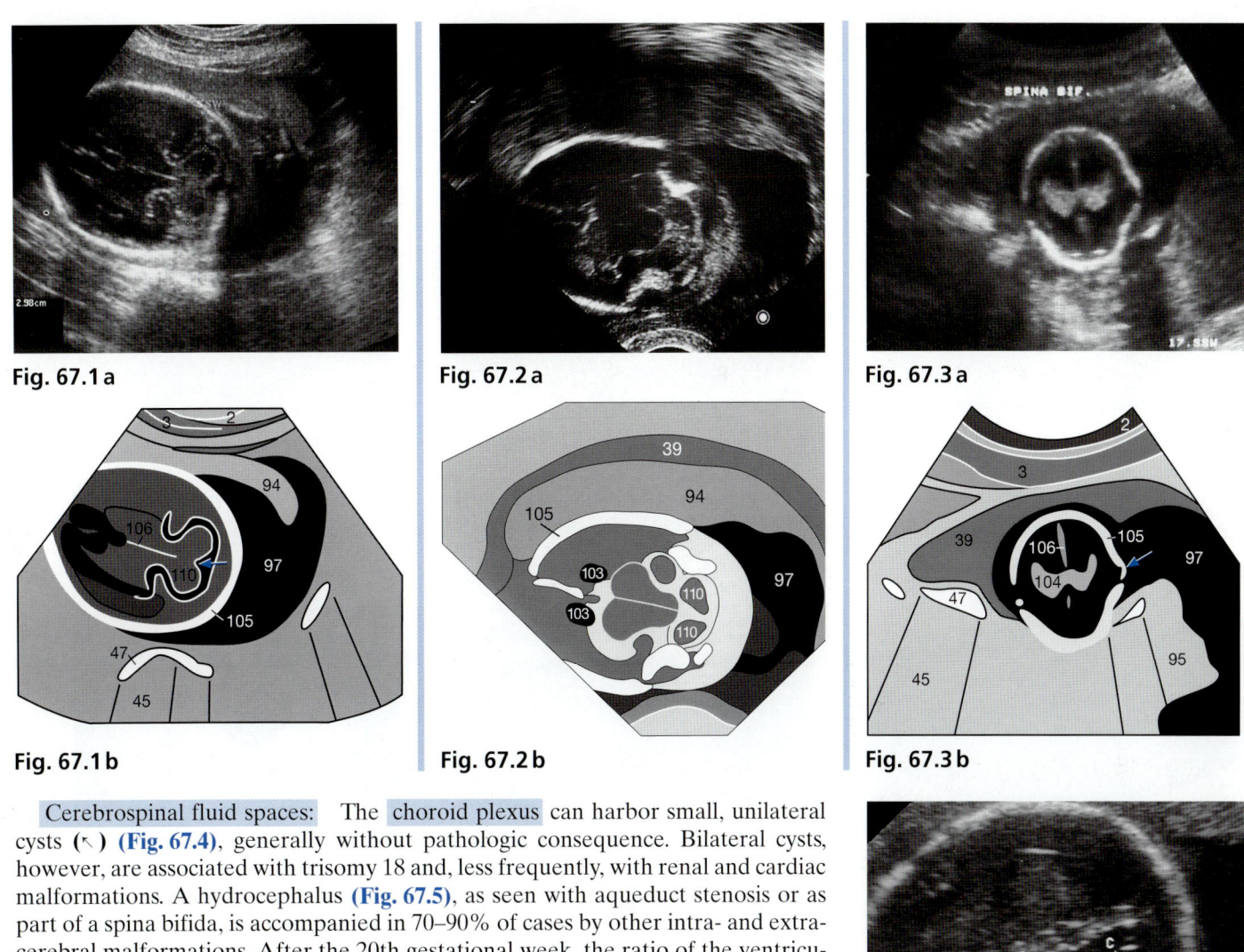

Fig. 67.1 a

Fig. 67.2 a

Fig. 67.3 a

Fig. 67.1 b

Fig. 67.2 b

Fig. 67.3 b

Cerebrospinal fluid spaces: The choroid plexus can harbor small, unilateral cysts (↖) (Fig. 67.4), generally without pathologic consequence. Bilateral cysts, however, are associated with trisomy 18 and, less frequently, with renal and cardiac malformations. A hydrocephalus (Fig. 67.5), as seen with aqueduct stenosis or as part of a spina bifida, is accompanied in 70–90% of cases by other intra- and extracerebral malformations. After the 20th gestational week, the ratio of the ventricular to the hemispheric diameter, also called the ventricular index, is used for assessing the ventricles, with a ratio of 0.5 considered indicative of hydrocephalus. The ratio at the level of the frontal horns (AHVR) is slightly exceeded by the ratio at the level of the occipital horn (PHVR) (Fig. 67.6 b). Measuring the diameter of the ventricles and hemispheres can be difficult because the lateral ventricular wall often is not clearly demarcated from the cerebral parenchyma (Fig. 67.6 a).

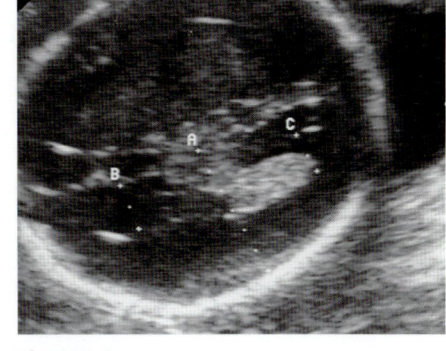

Fig. 67.6 a

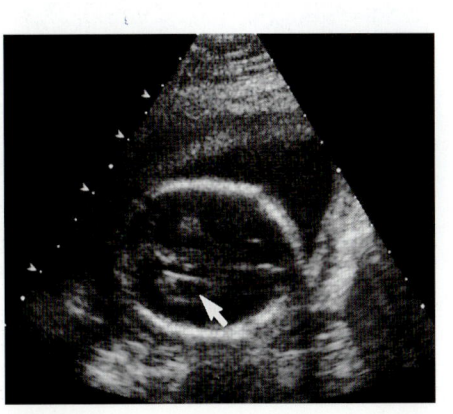

Fig. 67.4

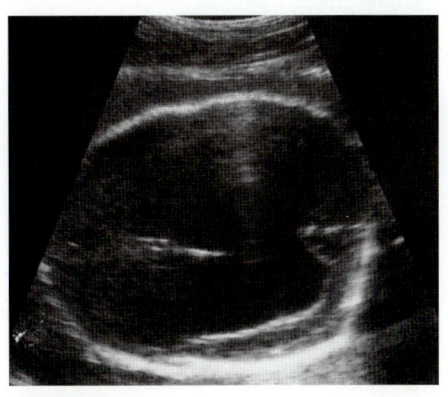

Fig. 67.5

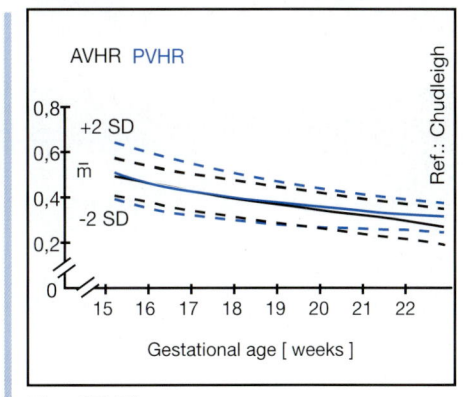

Fig. 67.6 b

11 Pregnancy — Diagnosis of Fetal Malformations

Spina bifida consists of incomplete closure of the spinal canal together with a defect in the spinal arches of varying degree. The spine **(35)** is visualized in the sagittal **(Fig. 68.1)** and coronal **(Fig. 68.2)** plane. Subsequently each vertebra is reviewed in the transverse plane in a craniocaudal direction since this will best reveal any interruption of the chain of the posterior elements, including the spinous process. The transverse section **(Fig. 68.3)** must delineate the three ossification centers **(35)** of each segment as a triangle of closely adjacent structures. The fetal aorta **(15)** is seen anteriorly.

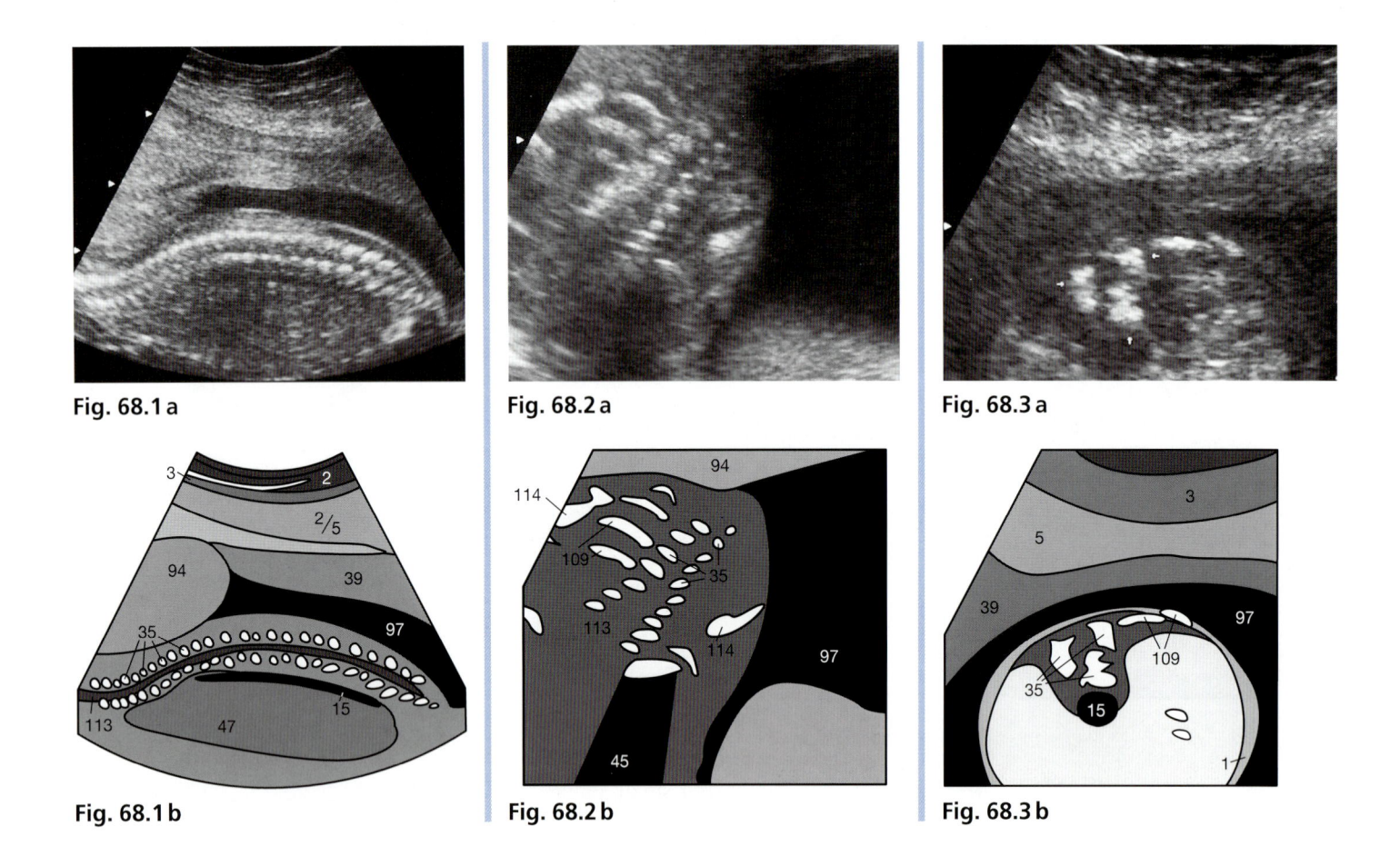

Fig. 68.1 a

Fig. 68.2 a

Fig. 68.3 a

Fig. 68.1 b

Fig. 68.2 b

Fig. 68.3 b

In spina bifida **(Fig. 68.4)**, both posterior ossification centers are splayed laterally and the spinal canal is dorsally open (↙↘). Measuring the maternal serum α-fetoprotein identifies only spina bifida aperta, but not the covered form, spina bifida occulta. The indirect sonographic signs of spina bifida ("banana" and "lemon" signs) have already been illustrated on page 67 **(refer to Figs. 67.2, 67.3)**.

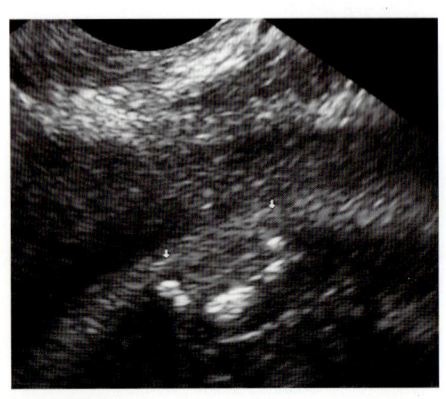

Fig. 68.4 a

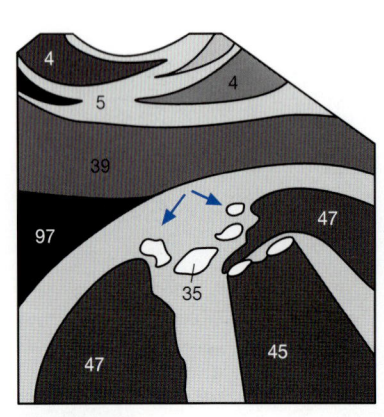

Fig. 68.4 b

11 Pregnancy — Diagnosis of Fetal Malformations

Facial bones and neck: Transverse and coronal sections of the face are usually evaluated for decreased (hypotelorism) or increased (hypertelorism) interorbital distance, and the sagittal sections for an atypical profile. A lip-palate cleft generally is lateral and can best be appreciated as a gap in the echogenic upper lip on the coronal section. The normal upper lip (→, ↘) appears as continuous structure **(Fig. 69.1)**.

Nuchal translucency (NT): After the 1st trimester, edema of the facial soft tissues or cervical subcutaneous tissue (hygroma colli) that *exceeds 3 mm* in width indicates imparied lymphatic drainage and in one third of cases it is associated with chromosomal abnormalities, such as monosomy X (Turner syndrome), trisomy 21 (Down syndrome), and trisomy 18. To distinguish a prominent nuchal membrane from an amniotic membrane along the posterior cervical area, the finding should be re-evaluated after fetal movements have been observed. Furthermore, a tangentially visualized cervical skin can mimic a double contour (↓) **(Fig. 69.2)**, which is invariably less than 3 mm in width. The more severe the elevation of the posterior cervical skin and the older the mother, the more likely a chromosomal abnormality **(Fig. 69.2 c)**.

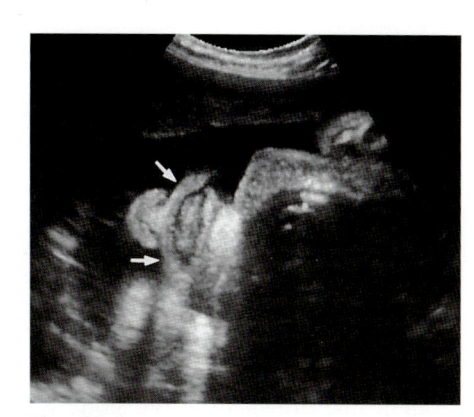

Fig. 69.1

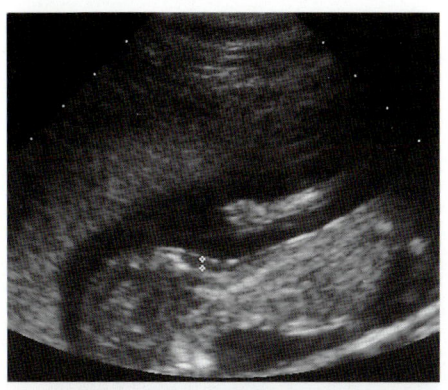

Fig. 69.2 a

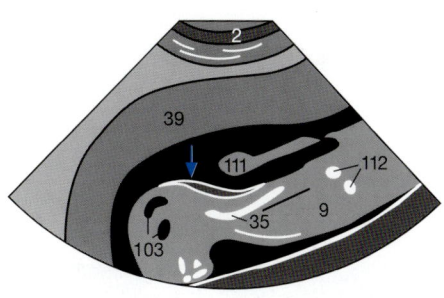

Fig. 69.2 b

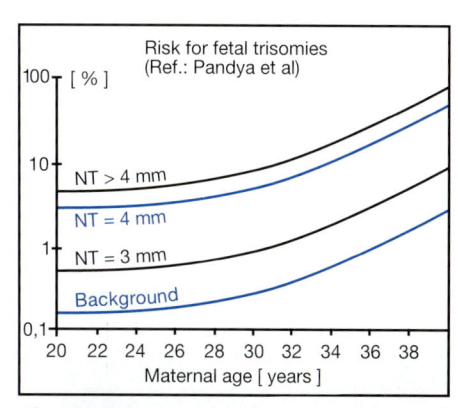

Fig. 69.2 c

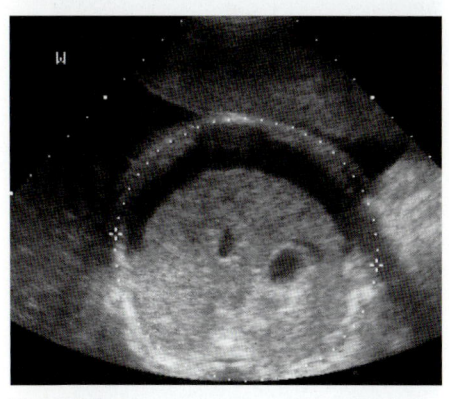

Hydrops fetalis: Increased fluid retention in serous cavities and placenta can be caused by cardiac insufficiency, metabolic disorder, infection-induced or congenital fetal anemia, rhesus immunization, and chromosomal abnormalities.

In monochorionic twins, the hydrops of one twin is caused by fetofetal transfusion through arteriovenous shunts.

In addition to showing an ascites (68) **(Fig. 69.3)**, sonography can visualize pleural and pericardial effusions (79) **(Fig. 69.4)** and possibly a generalized cutaneous edema.

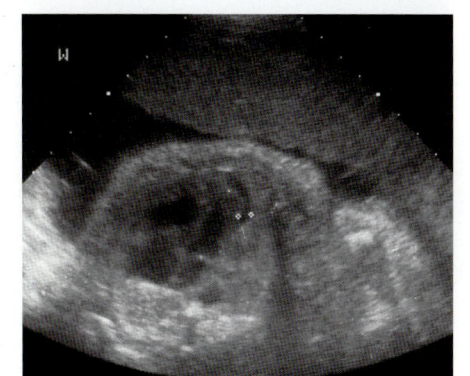

Fig. 69.3 a

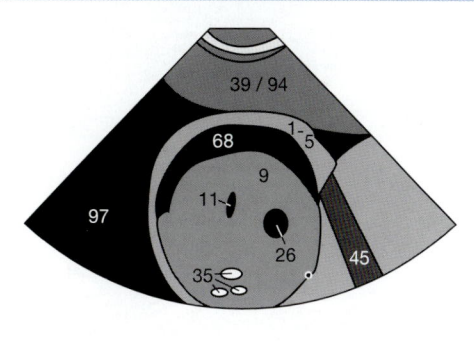

Fig. 69.3 b

Fig. 69.4 a

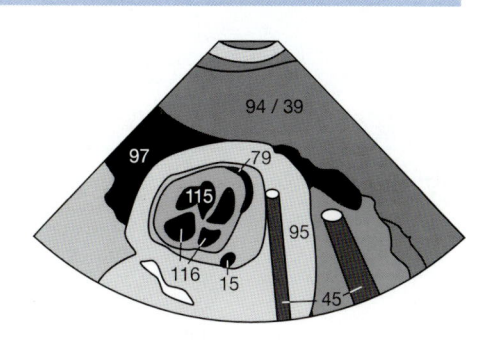

Fig. 69.4 b

11 Pregnancy — Diagnosis of Fetal Malformations

Heart and Vessels: The cardiovascular system is the first functioning organ system of the fetus. As from the 6th gestational week, fetal heart motion can be seen. Absent fetal heartbeats and growth retardation, usually accompanied by an indistinctly outlined fetus, indicate fetal demise and generally require dilatation and curettage. Because of their high sound energies, Doppler and color Doppler sonography should be used selectively, for instance, in cases of suspected growth retardation or cardiac malformation (refer to p. 63).

First, the position of the heart has to be determined: it should be one third to the right and two-thirds to the left of a straight line drawn from the spine to the anterior thoracic wall on the transverse section. The sagittal section must be oriented to visualize the aortic arch **(15)** and its brachiocephalic branches **(82, 117, 123)** **(Fig. 70.1)**. In addition to the cardiac valves, the four-chamber view should identify both atria **(116)** and both ventricles **(115)** **(Fig. 70.2)** and exclude any ventricular septum defect (VSD) or atrial septum defect (ASD). By tilting the probe slightly from this plane, the inflow of blood into the left ventricle through the mitral valve **(118)** as well as the outflow through the aortic valve **(119)** can be visualized in this so-called five-chamber view **(Fig. 70.3)**. Moreover, a VSD in the membranous portion of the septum is better delineated in this plane.

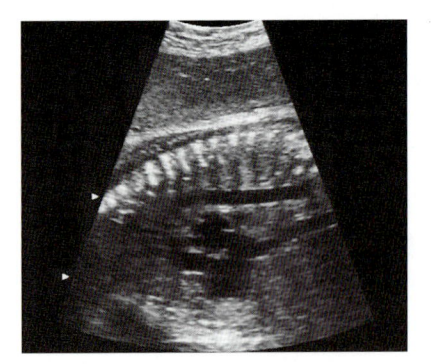

Fig. 70.1 a

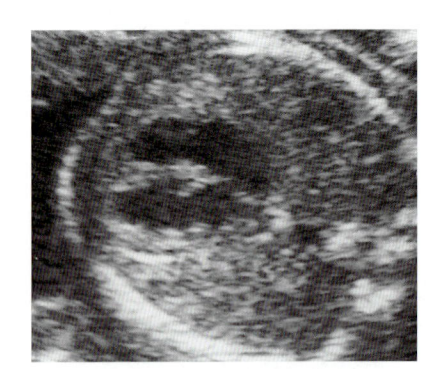

Fig. 70.2 a

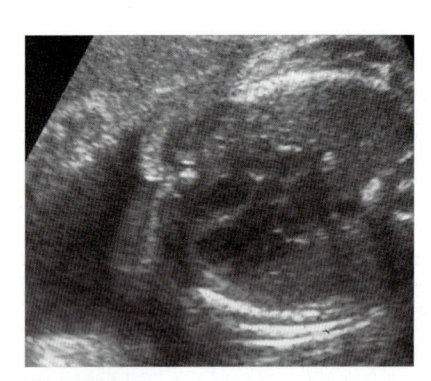

Fig. 70.3 a

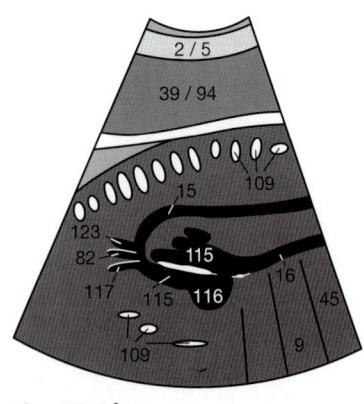

Fig. 70.1 b

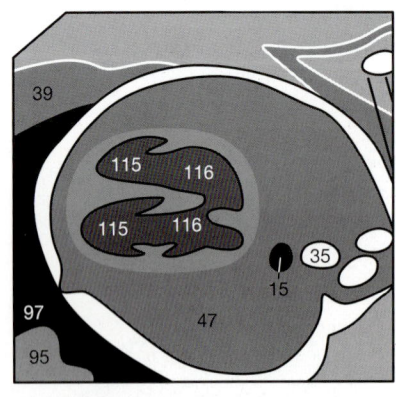

Fig. 70.2 b

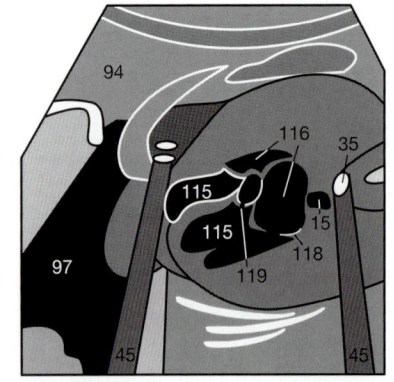

Fig. 70.3 b

A small ASD or VSD as well as cardiac anomalies with right-to-left shunts can be definitively excluded only by color-coded echocardiography performed by an experienced examiner. Transposition of the great arteries (TGA) might not be apparent on the four-chamber view and it is therefore necessary to look for crossed outflow tracts and aortic and pulmonic valves on the short axis view.

11 Pregnancy — Diagnosis of Fetal Malformations

The evaluation of the GI tract must, among other findings, exclude a "double bubble" sign, which would suggest a duodenal atresia or stenosis. The anechoic "bubbles" correspond to the stomach and to the duodenum proximal to the stenosis, respectively, both filled with fluid. This finding should be confirmed in a second plane, to avoid a false positive diagnosis due to double sectioning of the stomach in a tangential plane. It should be kept in mind that a hernia of the anterior abdominal wall **(120) (Fig. 71.1)** next to the umbilical vessels **(96)** is physiologic until the 11th gestational week and should not be mistaken for a true omphalocele.

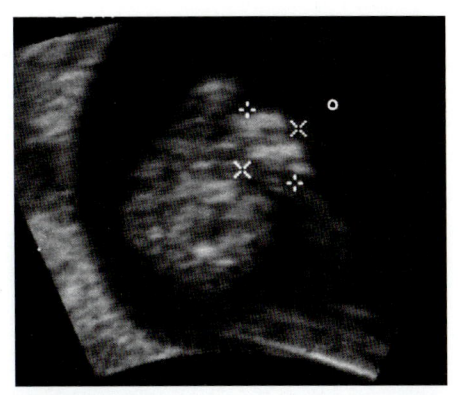

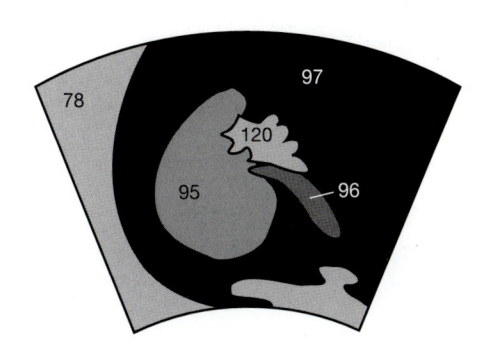

Fig. 71.1 a

Fig. 71.1 b

After the 15th gestational week, renal malformations are often indirectly revealed by a decreased amount of amniotic fluid (oligohydramnios) or its absence (anhydramnios) or by an empty urinary bladder because the amount of amniotic fluid corresponds to the renal excretion of urine at this time.

The normal renal parenchyma **(29)** already shows the less echogenic pyramids **(30)** separate from the anechoic collecting system **(31)** on the longitudinal section **(Fig. 71.2)**. A summary of the intrauterine growth of the kidney is found in **Figure 71.2 c**.

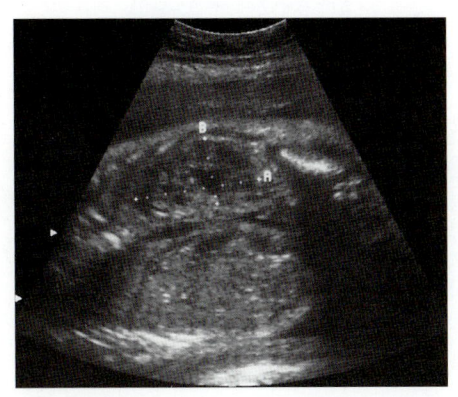

Fig. 71.2 a

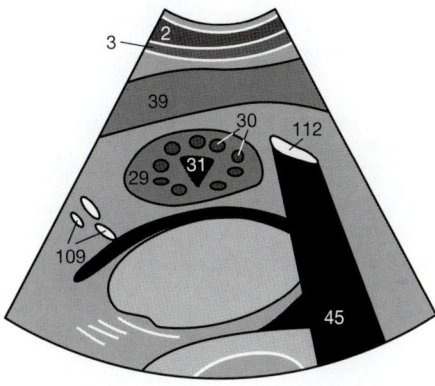

Fig. 71.2 b

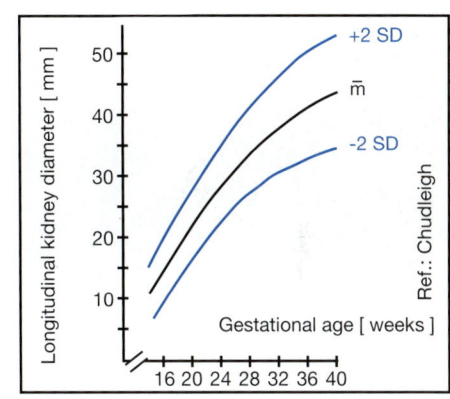

Fig. 71.2 c

Obstruction of the collecting system, as seen with ureteropelvic stenosis, is best recognized by comparing both sides on a transverse section through the renal hilum **(Fig. 71.3)**.

Polycystic renal disease becomes manifest in adulthood (type Potter III), prenatally as numerous visible renal cysts (type Potter II), or as a microcystic, hyperechoic kidney (type Potter I). Type Potter III polycystic renal disease might induce a prenatal, diffusely increased echogenicity, but this coexists with a normal amount of amniotic fluid and a filled urinary bladder.

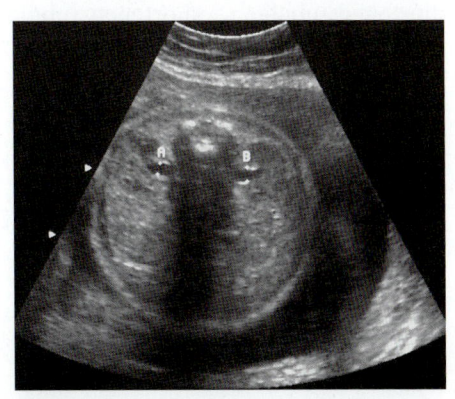

Fig. 71.3 a

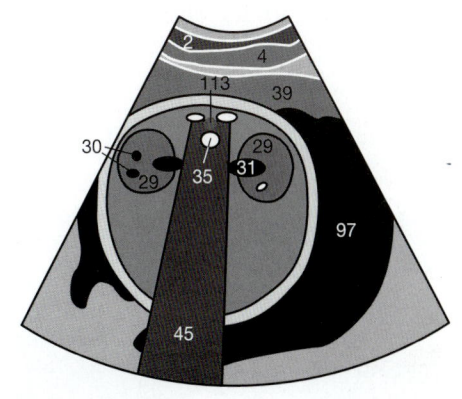

Fig. 71.3 b

11 Pregnancy — Diagnosis of Fetal Malformations

Skeletal System: In the second and third trimester, hands (Fig. 72.1) and feet (Fig. 72.2) are checked for complete development of the phalangeal ossification centers (121) and the metatarsal bones (122). In this way, syndactyly as part of other congenital malformation syndromes can be excluded.

Furthermore, supernumerous phalanges can be found, such as hexadactyly as seen in **Figure 72.3**. A polydactyly can be associated with shortened ribs and concomitant pulmonary hypoplasia. Not only are the shortened ribs apparent, but also the bell-shaped thorax.

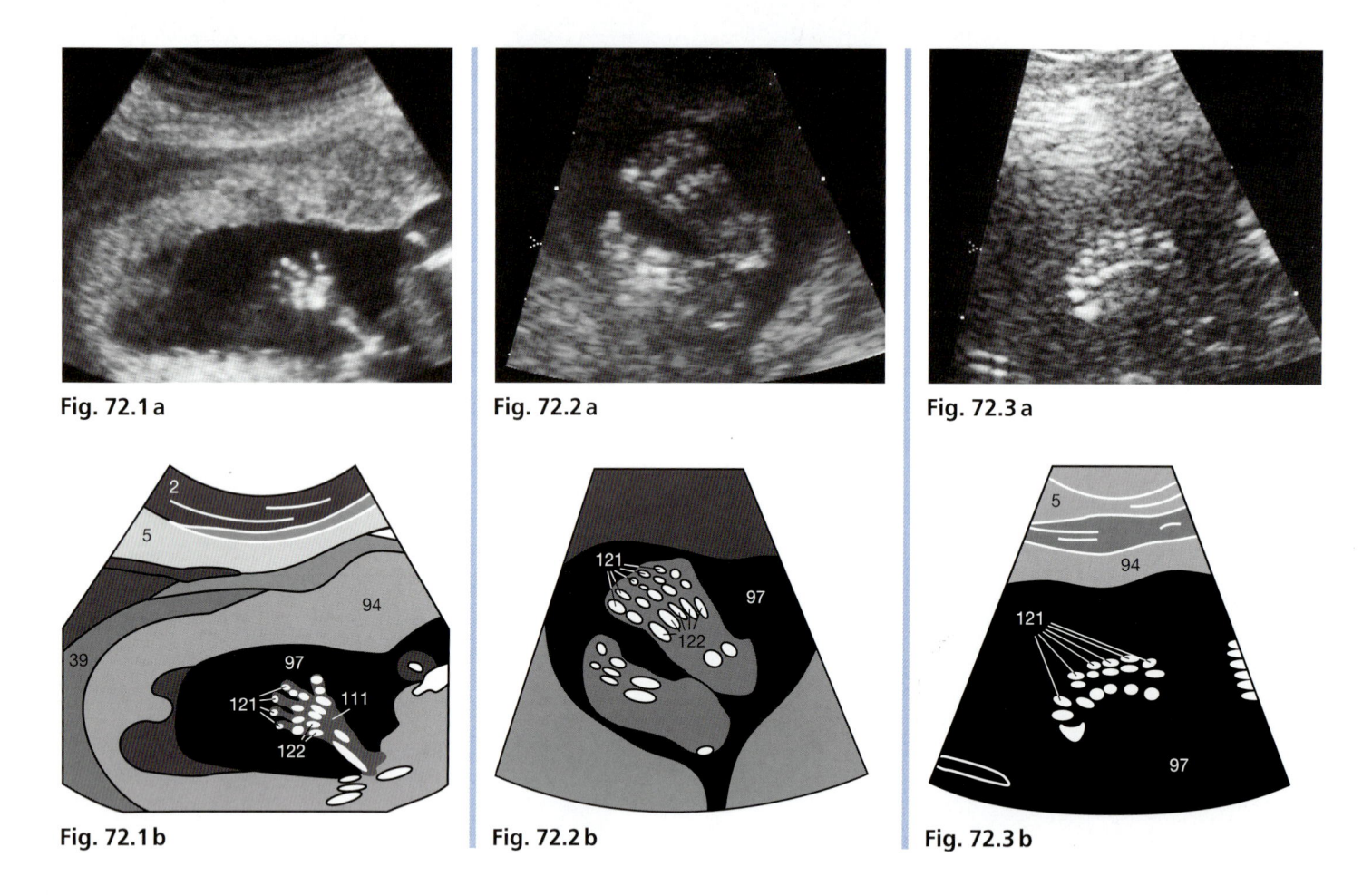

Fig. 72.1 a

Fig. 72.2 a

Fig. 72.3 a

Fig. 72.1 b

Fig. 72.2 b

Fig. 72.3 b

The search for a clubfoot anomaly should not be neglected (Fig. 72.4). The clubfoot does not only appear as a club-like deformity, but also as deviated shortened tubular bones.

Impaired enchondral ossification as part of achondroplasia is frequently recognized only in the 3rd trimester by shortened tubular bones and a head of disproportionately large appearence.

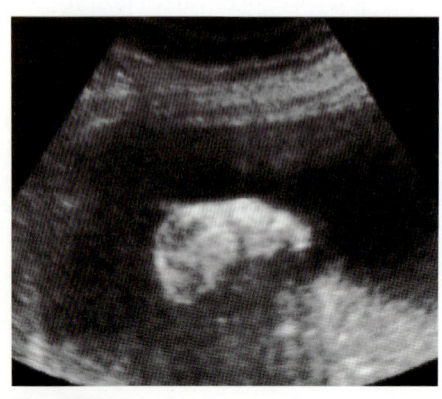

Fig. 72.4 a

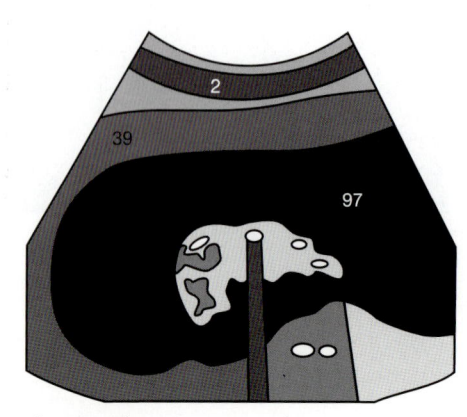

Fig. 72.4 b

11 Genitals and Prenatal Diagnosis — Questions for Self-Assessment

To conclude this section, you can again test how much detail you remember and how much still has to be memorized. The answers to question 1 and questions 3 to 6 can be found in the preceding pages, the answer to the quiz image of question 2 is given on page 77 at the end of the book.

1 An 18-year-old male patient presents with severe pain in the left scrotum, of sudden onset 3 hours ago and radiating into the left groin. What is your presumptive diagnosis? How much time do you have to proceed? What sonographic method do you select?

2 A 58-year-old female patient is referred to you for a sonographic evaluation of the pelvis. The patient had her menopause at the age of 52 years and currently does not take any hormone preparation. Endovaginal sonography produced the finding illustrated in **Figure 73.1**. The endometrium measures 18 mm in width. What diagnosis do you suspect and what measures do you initiate?

3 How do you recognize impending ovulation sonographically? What are the postovulatory changes? How many days after the last menstruation/after fertilization can the successful implantation be documented sonographically?

4 Write down the six biometric measurements next to this text. Add to each parameter the first and last gestational week of its meaningful application. At what gestational week is one parameter replaced by another parameter?

5 What are the direct and indirect sonographic criteria of spina bifida? Is a blood test of the mother sufficient?

6 What renal malformations do you know? Name at least three sonographic criteria.

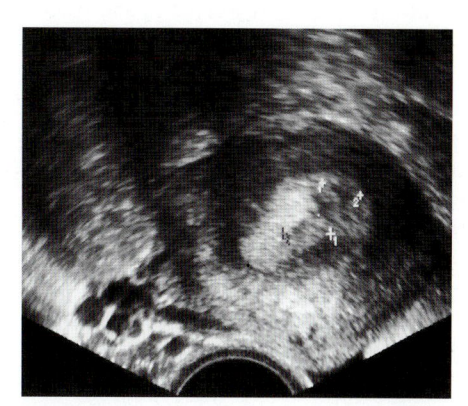

Fig. 73.1

Quiz for self-assessment

What is the imaging plane? Try to give a differential diagnosis for both cases. The answers can be looked up on page 77.

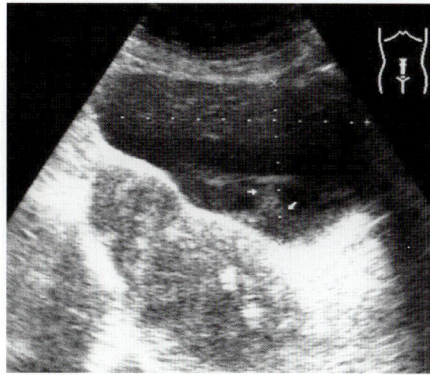

Fig. 73.2

Fig. 73.3

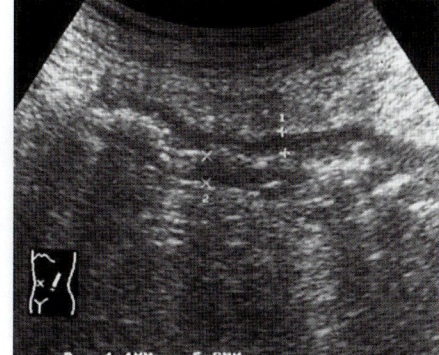

12 Thyroid Gland — Normal Findings

The thyroid gland is examined with a 7.5-MHz linear transducer. With the head slightly extended, transverse sections of the entire gland are obtained or, if the entire width of the gland cannot be encompassed, of each lobe separately (Fig. 74.1 a). Thereafter, sagittal sections are obtained through each thyroid lobe (Fig. 74.1 b). The trachea (84) with its air shadows in the midline and the carotid arteries (82) and jugular veins (83) with their echo-free lumina laterally serve as general orientation on the transverse sections. The thyroid parenchyma (81) is situated between the trachea and the vessels. Anterior to the trachea, a thin parenchymal band (isthmus) connects both thyroid lobes (compare Fig. 75.1).

With the patient performing a Valsalva maneuver (bearing down with the vocal chords closed), the jugular veins distend due to blocked venous drainage (Fig. 74.1 c). This makes orientation even easier.

The normal thyroid parenchyma (81) is slightly more echogenic than the anteriorly located sternohyoid muscle (89) and the more lateral sternocleidomastoid muscle (85). On cross section (Fig. 74.2), the carotid artery (82) is somewhat posteromedial in location and is visualized as a round noncompressible structure. In contrast, the jugular vein (83) runs more anterolaterally, exhibits a typical phasic pulse and can be compressed by applying graded (!) pressure. To assess the size of the thyroid gland, the maximum transverse and sagittal (anteroposterior) diameters of each lobe are measured on transverse sections (Fig. 74.2 b). Both values are multiplied by the maximum length as measured on the sagittal sections (Fig. 75.3 b) and are divided by two. Within an error range of approximately 10%, the result corresponds to the volume (in ml) of each lobe. Excluding the isthmus, which can be ignored because of its small size, the volume of the thyroid gland should not exceed 25 ml in men and 20 ml in women. Small thyroid cysts (64) might not cause any distal acoustic enhancement (Fig. 74.3) and must be differentiated from hypoechoic nodules (compare p. 75). Intrathyroidal vessels are rarely delineated.

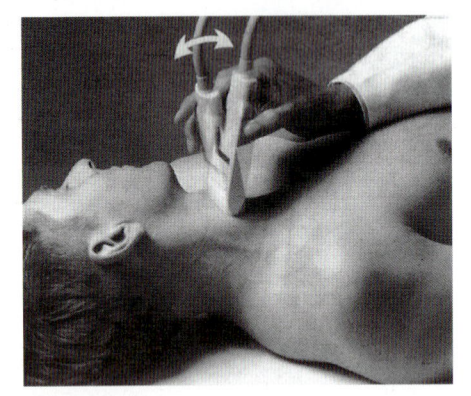

Fig. 74.1 a

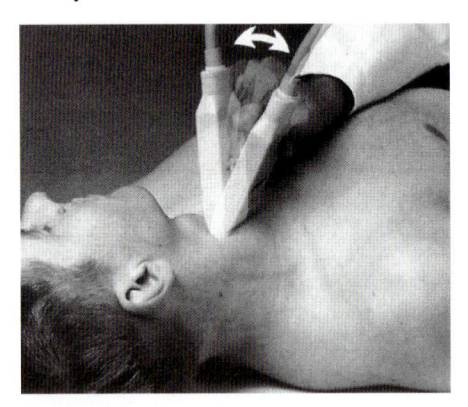

Fig. 74.1 b

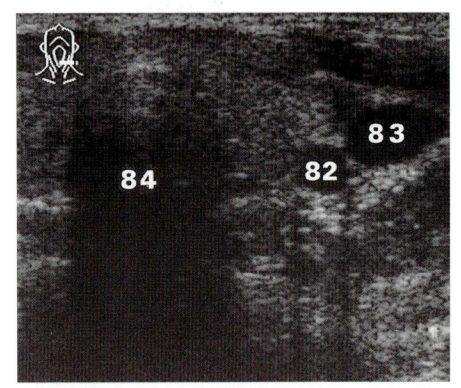

Fig. 74.1 c

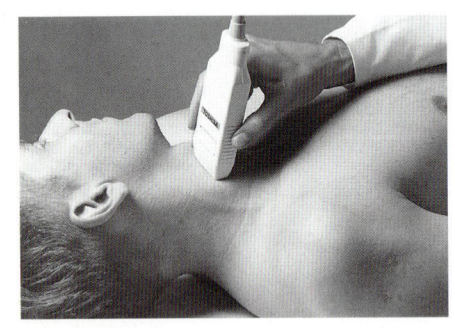

Fig. 74.2 a

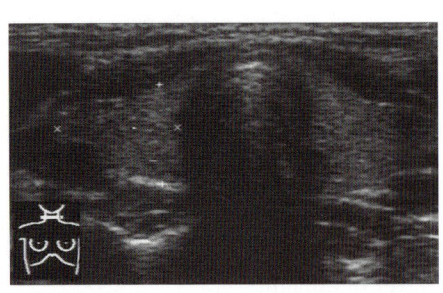

Fig. 74.2 b

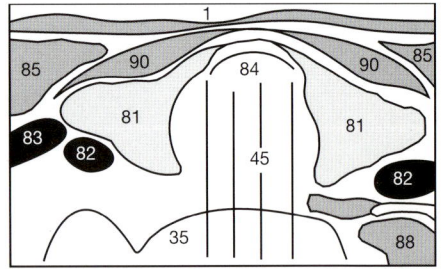

Fig. 74.2 c

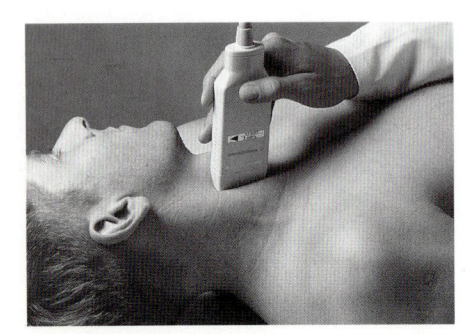

Fig. 74.3 a

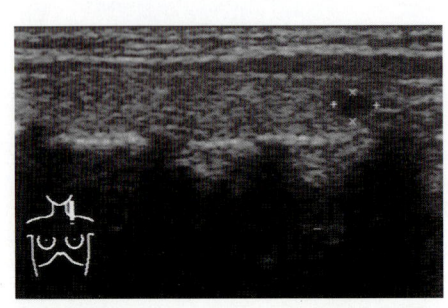

Fig. 74.3 b

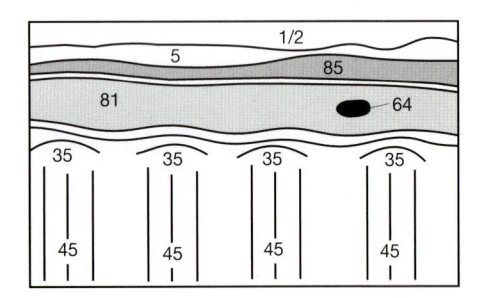

Fig. 74.3 c

Normal Measurements in Abdominal Ultrasonography in Children
(Adult measurements can be found on the back)

For liver and spleen, the **median values (m)** ± 2 SD in [cm] are related to body height and measured along the right and left median axillary line (not the MCL). The renal measurements [cm] are confidence intervals of the standard percentiles:

Body height [cm]	Liver m−2SD	Liver m	Liver m+2SD	Spleen m−2SD	Spleen m	Spleen m+2SD	Kidney 5%	Kidney 50%	Kidney 95%
Neonates	3.47	5.53	7.59	2.90	4.07	5.24	3.40	4.16	4.92
< 55	3.40	5.50	7.60	2.13	2.91	3.69	3.00	4.35	5.83
55– 70	4.53	6.59	8.65	2.44	3.46	4.48	3.60	5.00	6.40
71– 85	5.48	7.20	8.92	2.23	3.71	5.19	4.50	5.90	7.30
86–100	5.98	7.68	9.38	2.61	4.69	6.77	5.30	6.60	7.90
101–110	6.76	8.74	10.72	3.02	4.88	6.74	5.85	7.10	8.35
111–120	6.56	8.71	10.83	3.38	5.26	7.14	6.35	7.65	8.95
121–130	7.38	9.40	11.42	3.37	5.31	6.87	6.90	7.20	9.50
131–140	8.63	9.99	11.35	4.10	5.96	7.82	7.40	8.70	10.00
141–150	8.48	10.42	12.36	4.61	5.81	7.01	7.90	9.25	10.60
> 150	9.48	11.36	13.24	4.36	6.18	8.00	8.60	9.95	11.30

Ref.: Dinkel E et al: Kidney size in childhood, Pediatr Radiol (15): 38–43;
Weitzel D: Sonographische Organometrie im Kindesalter, Mainz

Normal Volumes of the Thyroid Gland [ml]
Both lobes combined, calculated according to the volume formula (0.5 × A × B × C).

Age	Girls m−1SD	Girls m	Girls m+1SD	Boys m−1SD	Boys m	Boys m+1SD
Neonates	0.5	1.1	1.7	0.4	1.2	2.0
< 1 Year	0.6	1.6	2.6	0.6	1.2	1.8
< 4 Years	1.6	2.4	3.2	1.0	1.7	2.4
< 8 Years	1.9	3.4	4.9	1.9	3.2	4.5
< 12 Years	3.2	5.7	8.2	3.5	5.7	7.9
> 12 Years	4.8	8.0	11.2	4.5	7.9	11.3
Adults		< 20			< 25	

Ref.: Peters H: Gehirn, in Deeg et al: Die Ultraschalluntersuchung des Kindes.
Springer Verlag, Berlin, Heidelberg, New York (1997): 443

Normal CSF Measurements in Neonates
- SCW (sinucortical width): ≤ 3 mm
- CCW (craniocerebral width): ≤ 4 mm
- IHW (Interhemispheric width): ≤ 6 mm
- Width of lateral ventricles (frontal horn): ≤ 13 mm

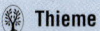

Thieme
Excerpt from:
Ultrasound Teaching Manual
ISBN 3 13 111041 4

Checklist of Criteria for Establishing a Cyst:
- Spherical configuration
- Echo-free interior
- Smooth outline
- Distal acoustic enhancement
- Sharply defined distal wall
- Edge shadowing due to critical angle phenomenon

Checklist of Criteria for Establishing Hepatic Cirrhosis:
- Absence of thin, hyperechoic capsular line
- Paucity of peripheral hepatic vessels
- Obtuse angulation of the hepatic veins > 45°
- Accentuated echogenic wall of the portal vein
- Abrupt caliber changes of the branches of the portal vein
- Regenerating nodules with displacement of adjacent vessels
- Nodular liver contour (advanced stage only)
- Contracted liver (advanced stage only)
- Signs of portal hypertension

Thieme
Excerpt from:
Ultrasound Teaching Manual
ISBN 3 13 111041 4

Normal Measurements in Prenatal Ultrasonography

Estimation of Fetal Weight

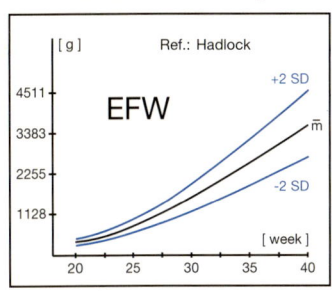

log FW = 1.36 + 0.05 AC + 0.18 FL − 0.0037 (AC × FL)

Ref.: Hadlock FB et al: Sonographic estimation of fetal weight. Radiology (1984): 536

FW = Fetal weight
AC = Abdominal circumference
FL = Femur length

Kidneys: Normal Weight

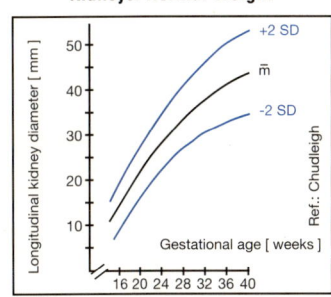

Ref.: Chudleigh P, Pearce JM: Obstetric Ultrasound; Churchill Livingstone (1992)

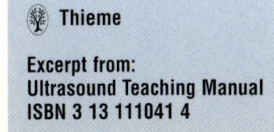

Thieme
Excerpt from:
Ultrasound Teaching Manual
ISBN 3 13 111041 4

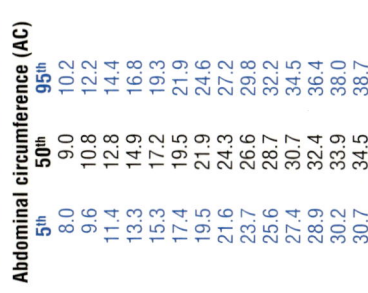

Normal Values in Prenatal Ultrasonography

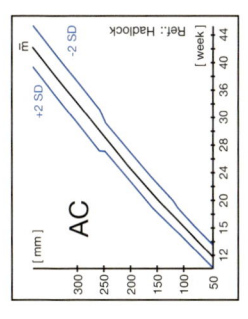

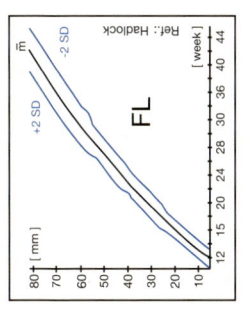

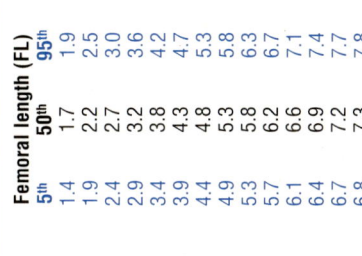

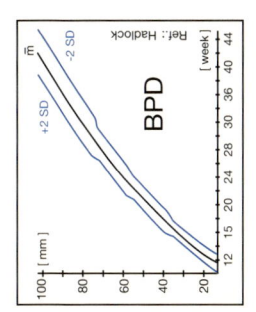

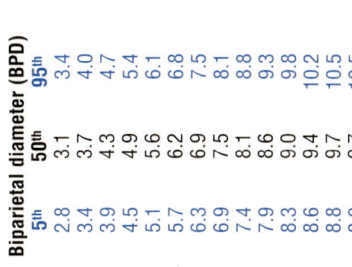

Abdominal circumference (AC)

Weeks	5th	50th	95th
14	8.0	9.0	10.2
16	9.6	10.8	12.2
18	11.4	12.8	14.4
20	13.3	14.9	16.8
22	15.3	17.2	19.3
24	17.4	19.5	21.9
26	19.5	21.9	24.6
28	21.6	24.3	27.2
30	23.7	26.6	29.8
32	25.6	28.7	32.2
34	27.4	30.7	34.5
36	28.9	32.4	36.4
38	30.2	33.9	38.0
39	30.7	34.5	38.7

Femoral length (FL)

Weeks	5th	50th	95th
14	1.4	1.7	1.9
16	1.9	2.2	2.5
18	2.4	2.7	3.0
20	2.9	3.2	3.6
22	3.4	3.8	4.2
24	3.9	4.3	4.7
26	4.4	4.8	5.3
28	4.9	5.3	5.8
30	5.3	5.8	6.3
32	5.7	6.2	6.7
34	6.1	6.6	7.1
36	6.4	6.9	7.4
38	6.7	7.2	7.7
39	6.8	7.3	7.8

Biparietal diameter (BPD)

Weeks	5th	50th	95th
14	2.8	3.1	3.4
16	3.4	3.7	4.0
18	3.9	4.3	4.7
20	4.5	4.9	5.4
22	5.1	5.6	6.1
24	5.7	6.2	6.8
26	6.3	6.9	7.5
28	6.9	7.5	8.1
30	7.4	8.1	8.8
32	7.9	8.6	9.3
34	8.3	9.0	9.8
36	8.6	9.4	10.2
38	8.8	9.7	10.5
39	8.9	9.7	10.5

Percentile values in [cm]; Ref.: Snijders RJM, Nicolaides KH: Ultrasound markers for fetal chromosomal defects, in: Frontiers in Fetal Medicine Series, The Parthenon Publishing Group, New York, London (1996): 174

Checklist Right Cardiac Insufficiency:

- Dilation of the inferior vena cava to > 2.0 cm (2.5 cm in trained athletes)
- Dilated hepatic vein > 6 mm in the hepatic periphery
- Absent caval collapse with forced inspiration
- Possible pleural effusion, initially almost always on the right

Checklist Aortic Aneurysm:

- Normal lumen: suprarenal < 2.5 cm
- Ectasia: 2.5–3.0 cm
- Aneurysm: > 3 cm
- Risk of rupture increased by: progressing dilation
  diameter > 6 cm
  excentric lumen
  saccular dilation (instead of fusiform dilation)

Checklist Portal Hypertension:

- Demonstration of portocaval collaterals at the porta hepatis
- Diameter of the portal vein at the porta hepatis > 15 mm
- Dilatation of the splenic vein > 1.2 cm
- Splenomegaly
- Demonstration of ascites
- Recanalized umbilical vein (Cruveilhier–Baumgarten syndrome)
- Esophageal varices (by endoscopy)

Normal Measurements in Abdominal Ultrasonography in Adults
(Pediatric measurements can be found on the back)

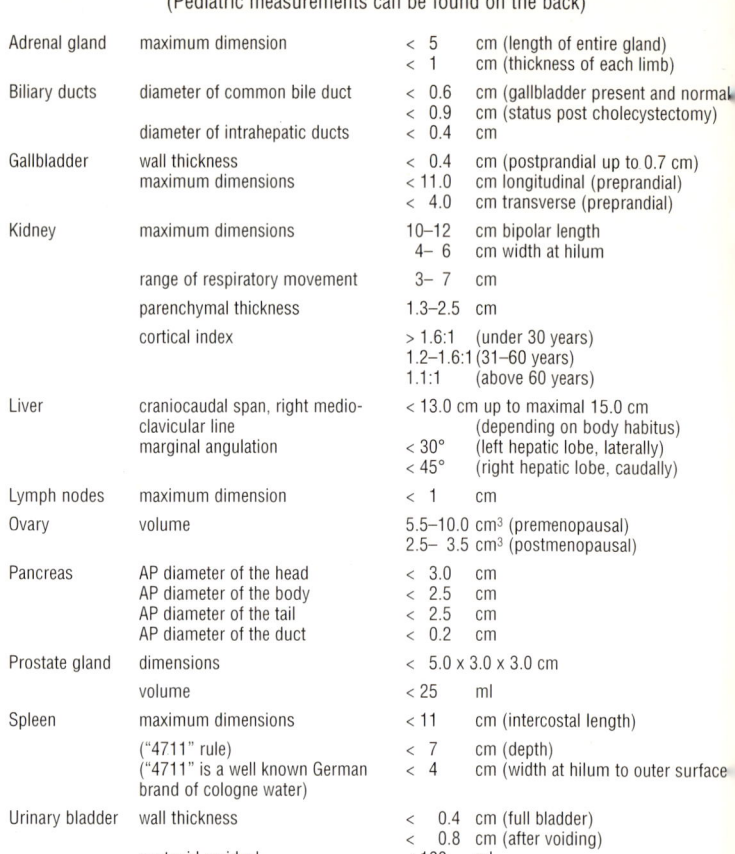

Adrenal gland	maximum dimension	< 5 cm	(length of entire gland)
		< 1 cm	(thickness of each limb)
Biliary ducts	diameter of common bile duct	< 0.6 cm	(gallbladder present and normal)
		< 0.9 cm	(status post cholecystectomy)
	diameter of intrahepatic ducts	< 0.4 cm	
Gallbladder	wall thickness	< 0.4 cm	(postprandial up to 0.7 cm)
	maximum dimensions	< 11.0 cm	longitudinal (preprandial)
		< 4.0 cm	transverse (preprandial)
Kidney	maximum dimensions	10–12 cm	bipolar length
		4–6 cm	width at hilum
	range of respiratory movement	3–7 cm	
	parenchymal thickness	1.3–2.5 cm	
	cortical index	> 1.6:1	(under 30 years)
		1.2–1.6:1	(31–60 years)
		1.1:1	(above 60 years)
Liver	craniocaudal span, right medioclavicular line	< 13.0 cm up to maximal 15.0 cm	(depending on body habitus)
	marginal angulation	< 30°	(left hepatic lobe, laterally)
		< 45°	(right hepatic lobe, caudally)
Lymph nodes	maximum dimension	< 1 cm	
Ovary	volume	5.5–10.0 cm^3	(premenopausal)
		2.5–3.5 cm^3	(postmenopausal)
Pancreas	AP diameter of the head	< 3.0 cm	
	AP diameter of the body	< 2.5 cm	
	AP diameter of the tail	< 2.5 cm	
	AP diameter of the duct	< 0.2 cm	
Prostate gland	dimensions	< 5.0 x 3.0 x 3.0 cm	
	volume	< 25 ml	
Spleen	maximum dimensions ("4711" rule)	< 11 cm	(intercostal length)
	("4711" is a well known German brand of cologne water)	< 7 cm	(depth)
		< 4 cm	(width at hilum to outer surface)
Urinary bladder	wall thickness	< 0.4 cm	(full bladder)
		< 0.8 cm	(after voiding)
	postvoid residual	< 100 ml	
	normal volume (A x B x C x 0.5)	< 550 ml	(females)
		< 750 ml	(males)
Uterus	maximum dimensions	5–8 cm	in length (nulliparous)
		1.5–3 cm	in width (nulliparous)
	endometrial width	< 15mm / < 8 mm	(pre-/postmenopausal)
	yolk sac	3.0–7.0 mm	
	IUD–fundus distance	< 20 mm	
	IUD–endometrium distance	< 5 mm	

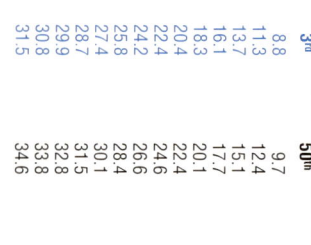

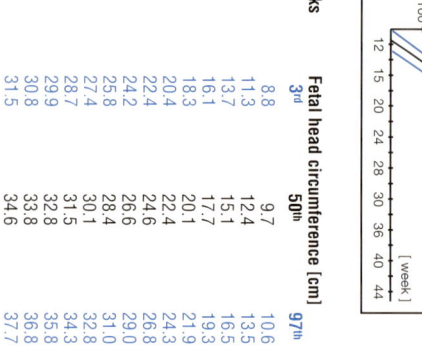

Normal Values in Prenatal Ultrasonography

Gestational sac diameter (GSD) — n = 2262, Ref.: Holzgreve

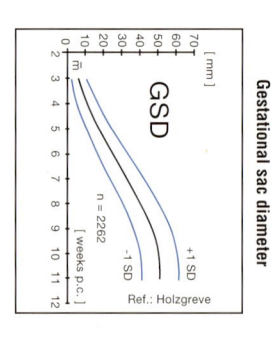

Week	GSD	Week	GSD	Week	GSD	Week	GSD
5.0	1.0		2.7		4.4		
5.2	1.1		2.8		4.5		
5.3	1.2		2.9		4.6		
5.5	1.3		3.0		4.7		
5.6	1.4		3.1		4.8		
5.8	1.5		3.2		4.9		
5.9	1.6		3.3		5.0		
6.0	1.7		3.4		5.1		
6.2	1.8		3.5		5.2		
6.3	1.9		3.6		5.3		
6.5	2.0		3.7		5.4		
6.6	2.1		3.8		5.5		
6.8	2.2		3.9		5.6		
6.9	2.3		4.0		5.7		
7.0	2.4		4.1		5.8		
7.2	2.5		4.2		5.9		
7.3	2.6		4.3		6.0		

(mean values in [cm]; Ref.: Hellman et al, Am J Obstet Gynecol (1969);103:789)

Yolk sac diameter (YSD) — Ref.: Holzgreve

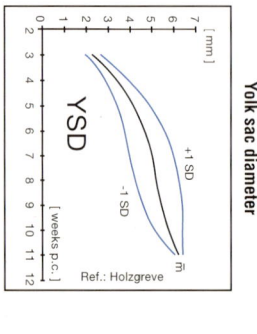

Crown-rump-length (CRL) — Ref.: Hadlock

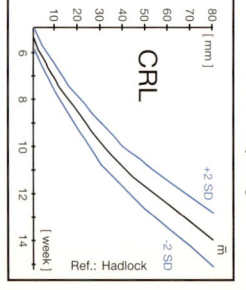

Week	CRL	Week	CRL	Week	CRL
5+5	1.2			5+6	2.1
6+6	8.5		23.5	10+6	41.3

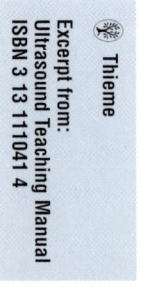

(mean values in [mm]; Ref.: Rempen)

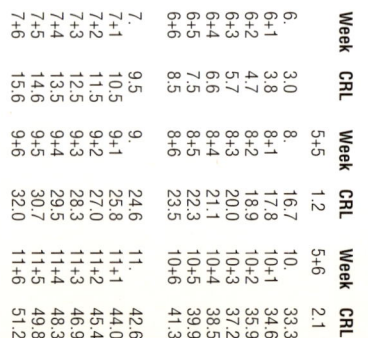

Fetal head circumference [cm] (3rd, 50th, 97th percentile)

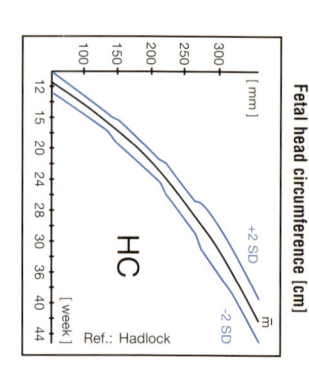

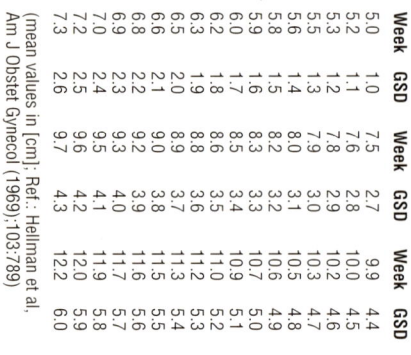

Weeks	3rd	50th	97th
14	8.8	9.7	10.6
16	11.3	12.4	13.5
18	13.7	15.1	16.5
20	16.1	17.7	19.3
22	18.3	20.1	21.9
24	20.4	22.4	24.3
26	22.4	24.6	26.8
28	24.2	26.6	29.0
30	25.8	28.4	31.0
32	27.4	30.1	32.8
34	28.7	31.5	34.3
36	29.9	32.8	35.8
38	30.8	33.8	36.8
40	31.5	34.6	37.7

Fetal head circumference (HC) — Ref.: Hadlock

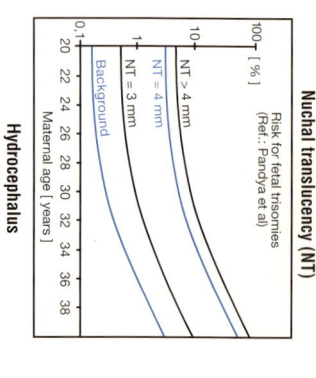

Hydrocephalus 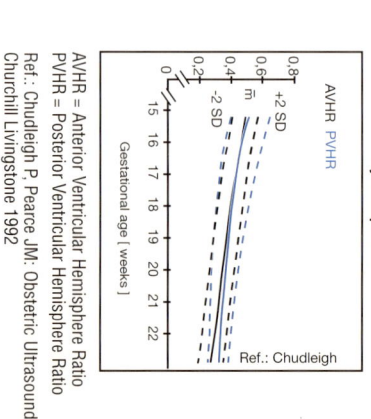 — AVHR = Anterior Ventricular Hemisphere Ratio; PVHR = Posterior Ventricular Hemisphere Ratio. Ref.: Chudleigh P, Pearce JM: Obstetric Ultrasound; Churchill Livingstone 1992

Nuchal translucency (NT) — Risk for fetal trisomies (Ref.: Pandya et al)

Excerpt from:
Ultrasound Teaching Manual
ISBN 3 13 111041 4

Thieme

12 Thyroid Gland — Diffuse and Focal Changes

The most common diffuse thyroid condition is iodine deficiency goiter. The thyroid gland **(81)** is diffusely enlarged and its echogenicity is slightly enhanced **(Fig. 75.2)**. A homogeneous hypoechogenicity (the thyroid gland has become iso-echoic with the musculature) is characteristic of Graves disease or inflammatory conditions such as Hashimoto thyroiditis.

Focal changes have to be separated into benign cysts **(64)** and solid lesions **(Fig. 75.3)**, by employing the usual criteria that establish a cyst (compare p. 29). Solid lesions comprise adenomas **(54)** as seen in **Figure 75.4** and nodular degenerative changes as well as malignant processes.

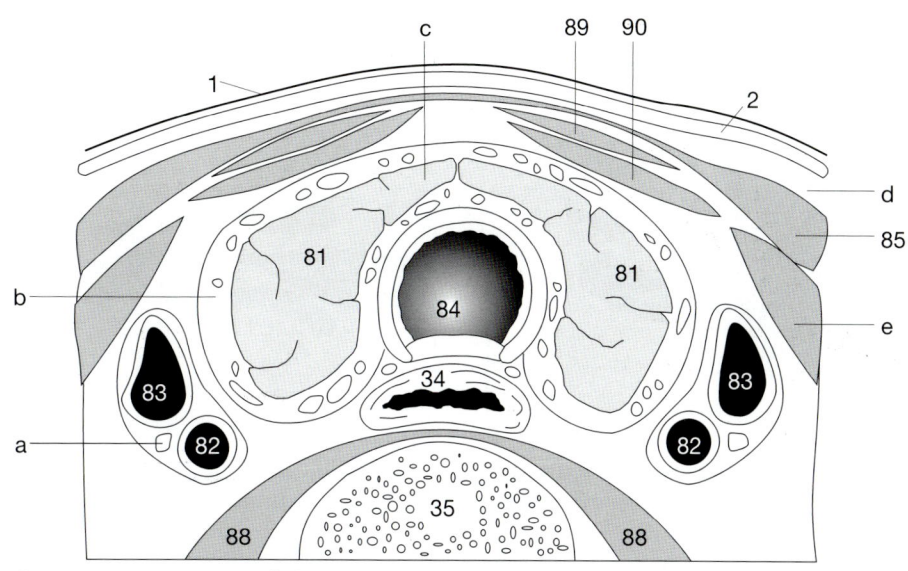

Fig. 75.1 Anatomy of the thyroid region.
Vagus nerve (a), fibrous capsule of thyroid (b), isthmus (c), platysma (d), omohyoid muscle (e), skin (1), subcutaneous fat tissue (2), esophagus (34), spine (35), lateral lobes of thyroid (81), common carotid artery (82), internal jugular vein (83), trachea (84), sternocleidomastoid muscle (85), anterior and medial scalenus muscles (88), sternohyoid muscle (89), sternothyroid muscle (90).

Frequently, calcifications are encountered in the thyroid parenchyma, generally representing areas of degenerative or postinflammatory regression that do not require further evaluation.

The decisive information for further assessment of a hypoechoic nodule is provided by the radionuclide thyroid scan because the functional status of a nodule cannot be deduced from its sonographic features. Scintigraphically functioning nodules ("hot" nodules) primarily correspond to areas of adenomatous hyperplasia or true adenomas, whereas non-functioning hypoechoic nodules ("cold" nodules) must arouse suspicion of malignancy and are generally subjected to sonographically-guided needle aspiration biopsy.

Though hyperechoic nodules are less likely to be malignant, they also should be considered for needle aspiration biopsy, unless their true nature can be established by combining the results of laboratory tests, sonography, and scintigraphy.

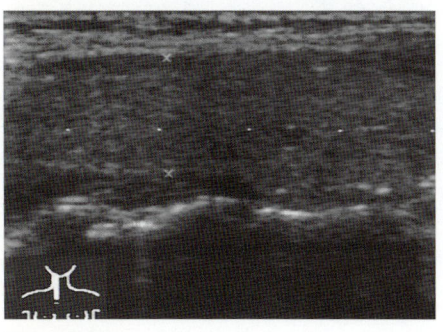

Fig. 75.2 a

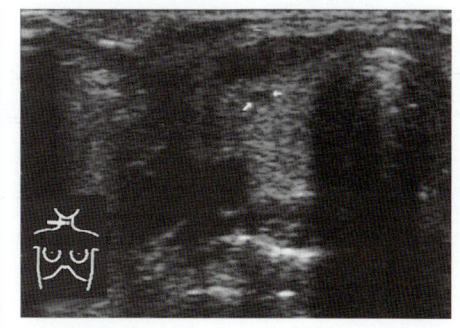

Fig. 75.3 a

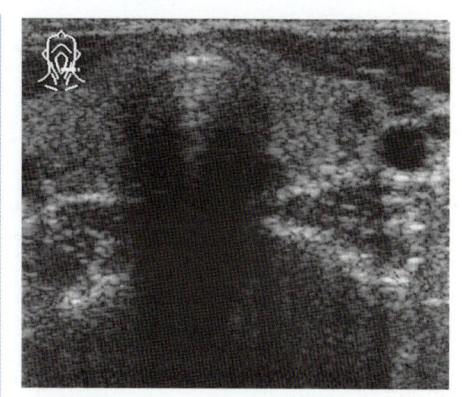

Fig. 75.4 a

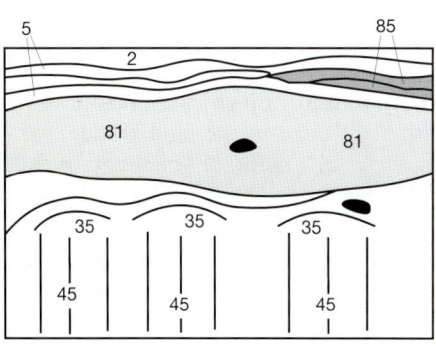

Fig. 75.2 b

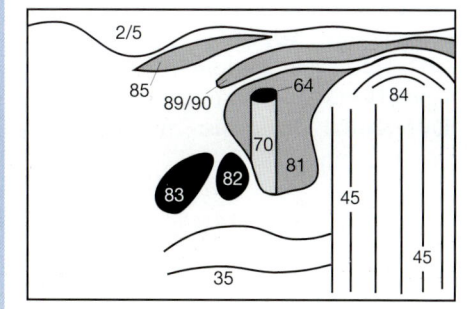

Fig. 75.3 b

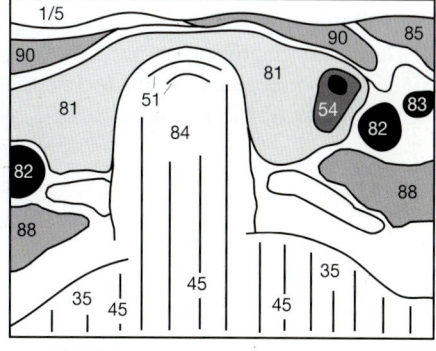

Fig. 75.4 b

Solutions to the Quiz

Solution to Fig. 16.2 (question 7):

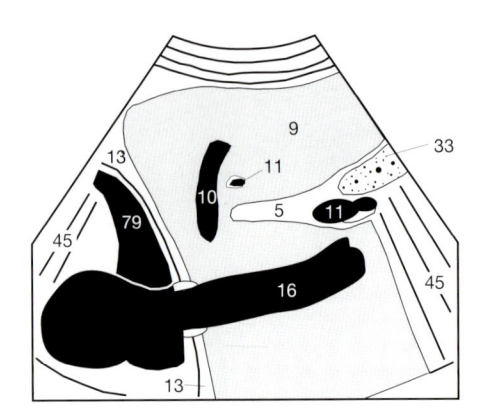

Sonographic section: sagittal section of the upper abdomen, paramedian over the inferior vena cava **(16)**.
Organs: liver **(9)**, heart, and pancreas **(33)**.
Structures: diaphragm **(13)**, hepatic veins **(10)**, portal branch **(11)**, connective tissue **(5)**, caudate lobe between 5 and 16.
Abnormal finding: echo-free space between the myocardium and diaphragm.
Diagnosis: pericardial effusion **(79)**.
Differential diagnosis: epicardial fat.

Solution to Fig. 22.1 (question 4):

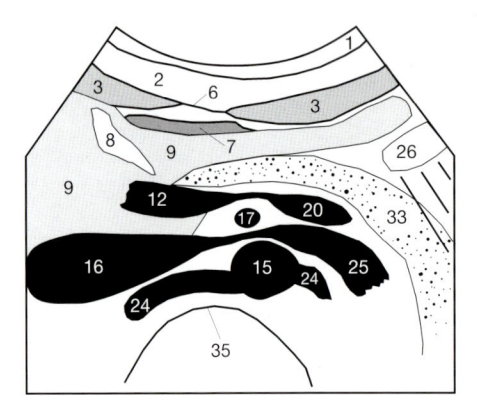

Sonographic section: sagittal section of the upper abdomen at the level of the left renal vein crossing the aorta.
Vessels and structures: refer to key on the unfolded back cover.
Dilatation?: no, only dilated left renal vein due to compression between aorta **(15)** and SMA **(17)**, still physiologic.

Solution to Fig. 33.1 (question 6):

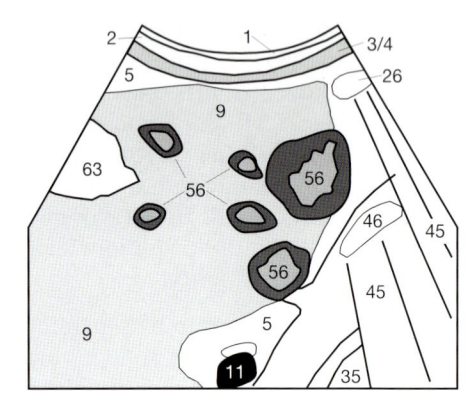

Sonographic section: oblique subcostal section of the right upper quadrant of the abdomen.
Diagnosis: Focal fatty infiltration **(63)** of the liver **(9)** and multiple hepatic metastases **(56)** with hypoechoic rim. Note: two episodes of metastatic spreading since new and older metastatic foci are visible!
Differential diagnosis: none, the finding is pathognomonic.

Solution to Fig. 33.2 (question 6):

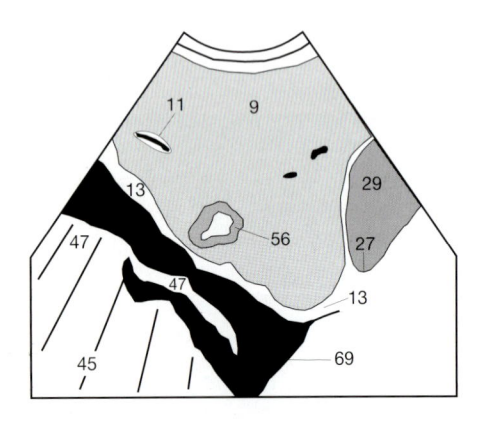

Sonographic section: sagittal section along the right MCL.
Diagnosis: subdiaphragmatic hepatic metastasis **(56)** with hypoechoic rim, pleural effusion **(69)**.
Differential diagnosis: hemangioma instead of a metastasis considering the echogenicity of the lesion.

Solution to Fig. 33.3 (question 6):

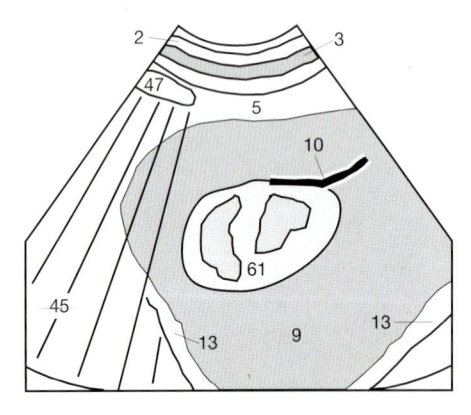

Sonographic section: sagittal section of the right upper quadrant of the abdomen along the paramedian plane.
Diagnosis: Hyperechoic, partially heterogeneous space-occupying lesion **(61)**. Here: hemangioma with draining vein **(10)** arising from it.
Differential diagnosis: tumor, hyperechoic metastasis.

Solution to Fig. 36.3 (question 2):

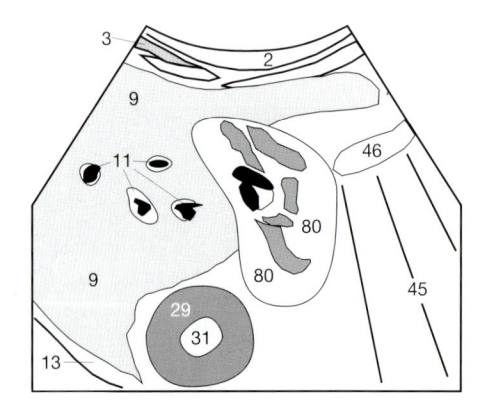

Sonographic section: oblique subcostal section of the right upper quadrant of the abdomen, liver **(9)**.
Diagnosis: cholecystitis with markedly thickened wall **(80)**.
Differential diagnosis: postprandial biliary sludge in the gallbladder, parasitic involvement of the liver or gallbladder.

Solutions to the Quiz

Solution to Fig. 46.1 (question 6):

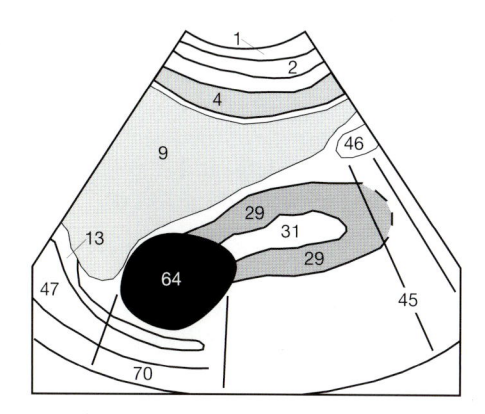

Sonographic section: intercostal plane of the right flank in left lateral decubitus position.
Organs: liver (9), renal parenchyma (29) with renal pelvis (31), lung (47), abdominal oblique musculature (4), diaphragm (13), intestinal loop (46).
Diagnosis: renal cyst (64) with distal acoustic enhancement (70).
Differential diagnosis: adrenal tumor with cystic component.

Solution to Fig. 46.2 (question 6):

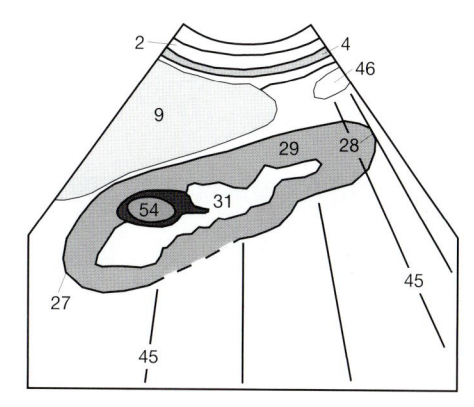

Sonographic section: intercostal plane of the right flank in left lateral decubitus position.
Organs: liver (9), abdominal oblique vasculature (4), interstinal loop (46) with acoustic shadowing (45), renal parenchyma (29), renal pelvis (31), upper renal pole (27), lower renal pole (28).
Diagnosis: renal cell carcinoma (54), hypoechoic tumor with space-occupying effect.
Differential diagnosis: renal lymphoma, metastasis, hyperplastic column of Bertin, hemorrhagic renal cyst.

Solution to Fig. 50.1 (question 5):

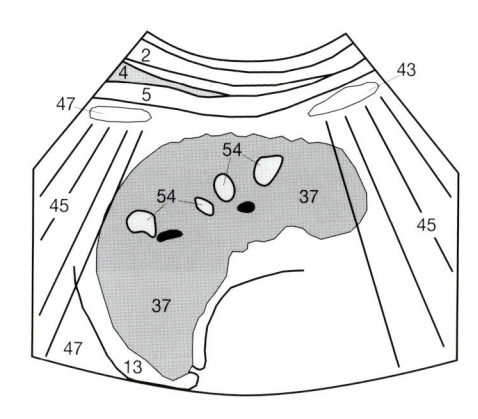

Sonographic section: high section of the left flank in the right lateral decubitus position.
Organs: spleen (37), lung (47), colon (43), diaphragm (13).
Parenchyma: not normally homogeneous, but patchy with several interspersed hyperechoic foci.
Diagnosis: multiple splenic hemangiomas.
Differential diagnosis: hyperechoic metastases, vasculitis due to SLE, histiocytosis X.

Solution to Fig. 73.1 (question 2):

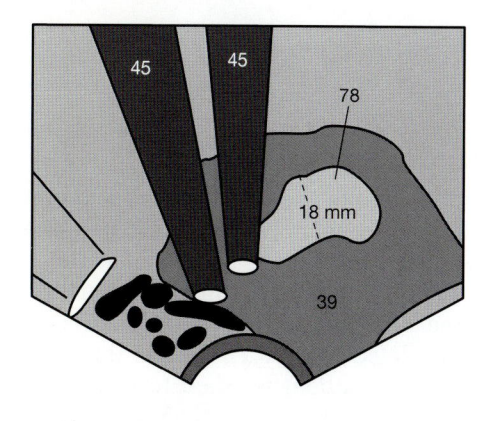

Imaging plane: endovaginal visualization of the uterus.
Diagnosis: endometrial hyperplasia (78) >8 mm in a postmenopausal woman *without* estrogen replacement therapy (refer to question).
Recommendation: fractionated dilatation and curettage to exclude an endometrial carcinoma.

Solution to Fig. 73.2:

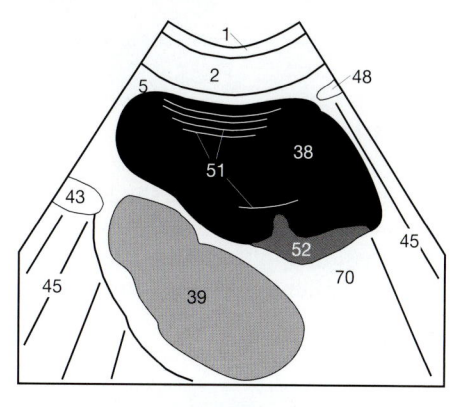

Sonographic Section: suprapubic longitudinal (sagittal) section of the lower abdomen.
Organs: urinary bladder (38), uterus (39, intestinal loop (43).
Diagnosis: blood clot (52) layered along the posterior wall of the urinary bladder.
Differential Diagnosis: Arch artifacts (51) and reverberation echoes (51) in the anterior aspect of the urinary bladder; layered concrements, thickness artifacts ⟶ shaking!

Solution to Fig. 73.3:

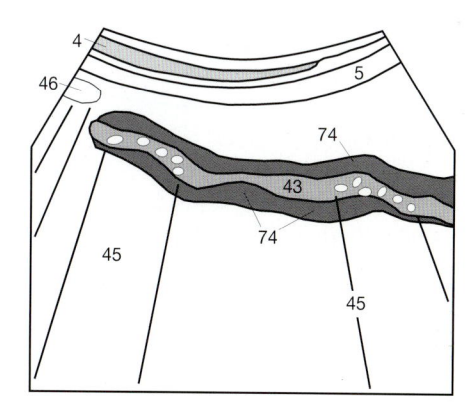

Sonographic Section: oblique section of the left lower quadrant of the abdomen.
Organs: abdoimal oblique muscles (4), colon (43).
Diagnosis: multilayered wall-thickening caused by colitis.
Differential Diagnosis: ischemia of the intestinal wall caused by thrombosis of the mesenteric vein or occlusion of the mesenteric artery.

Tips and Tricks for the Beginner

In preparation for the practical sections, the student should become familiar with the spatial orientation in a three-dimensional space. As an introduction, only two planes that are perpendicular to each other should be considered: the vertical (sagittal) plane and the horizontal (transverse) plane. As suggested on page 4, a cone coffee filter should be used to envisage how the sound waves in these two planes propagate from the transducer through the body.

All sagittal sections are conventionally viewed as seen from the patient's right side (Fig. 78.1 b). Consequently, the cranial aspect of the patient is displayed on the left and the caudal aspect on the right (Fig. 78.1 d).

After turning the transducer 90° (Fig. 78.1 d), the sonographic cross sections, like axial CT sections, are viewed from the patient's feet, resulting in an inverted display of the visualized structures (Fig. 78.1 c). What both sections have in common is that the image displays the anterior abdominal wall, including transducer, on the top and the posterior structures on the bottom. This orientation conforms to the customary display of conventional radiographs, CT, and MRI. Standing in front of the patient, the liver, for instance, is seen on the left though in actual fact it is on the patient's right side.

Sagittal views:

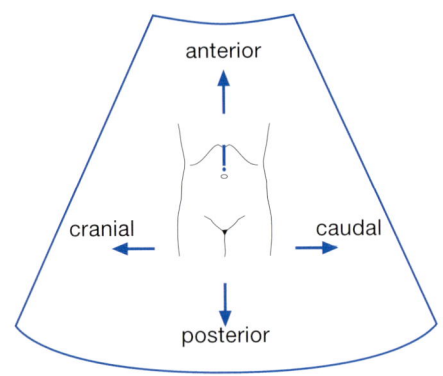

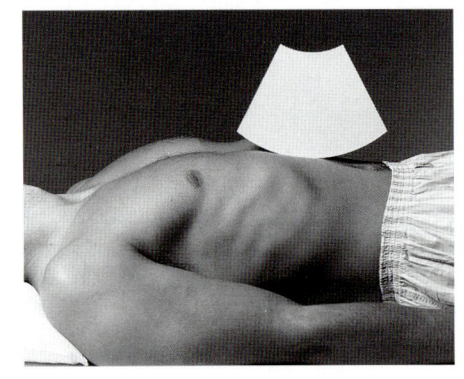

Fig. 78.1 a

Fig. 78.1 b

Transversal views:

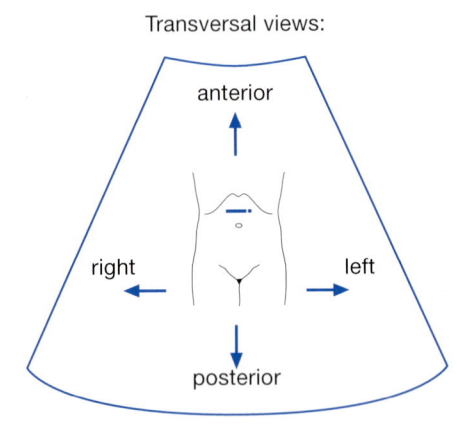

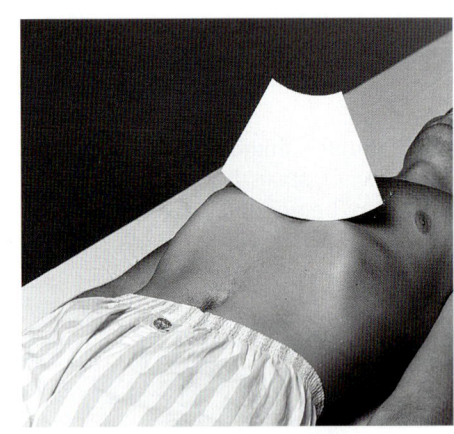

Fig. 78.1 c

Fig. 78.1 d

The next difficulty consists of visualizing structures amidst acoustic shadows cast by intestinal air. The solution is not the addition of more coupling gel, as the novice often believes, but a graded increase in the pressure applied to the transducer together with proper breathing instructions for the patient, explained further and illustrated on the next page.

If, despite every maneuver, the porta hepatis could not be visualized because of meteorism or a postprandial state, an attempt should be made to visualize the porta hepatis intercostally through the liver (Fig. 78.2). Should this also fail, the patient is asked to turn onto the left side and to continue turning beyond the lateral decubitus position (Fig. 78.3). The liver is pushed by its own weight against the anterior abdominal wall and displaces the air-containing intestinal loops laterally. This frequently opens up the view for the portal vein and lesser omentum.

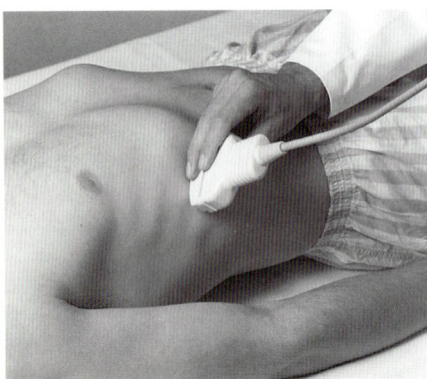

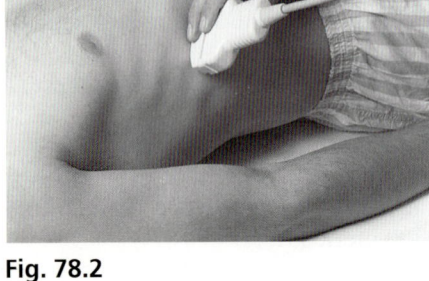

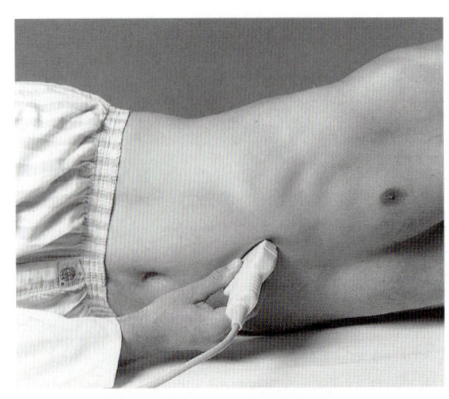

Fig. 78.2

Fig. 78.3

Tips and Tricks for the Beginner

Optimal adaption of the pressure on the transducer

To avoid any patient discomfort, the beginner is often reluctant to press the transducer firmly on to the abdomen. If this is the case (↓ ↓ ↓), physiologic air remains in the intestinal lumen (46), causing acoustic shadowing (45) that can, for instance, interfere with visualizing the posteriorly located pancreas (33) **(Fig. 79.1 a)**. Even the bile duct (66) or the portal vein (11) is frequently obscured by duodenal air or an air-distended stomach.

The solution lies in increasing the pressure applied to the transducer (↓↓↓), but the increase should be gradual rather than sudden to avoid any defense reflex or antagonistic reaction by the patient. By carefully displacing the intestinal air, this maneuver displaces the interfering air shadows (45), and the pancreas (33) and common bile duct (66) come into view **(Fig. 79.1 b)**. The same principle can be applied to the mid and lower abdomen, for instance, for improving the visualization of retroperitoneal lymph nodes.

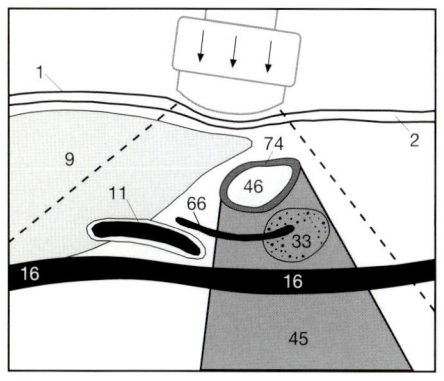

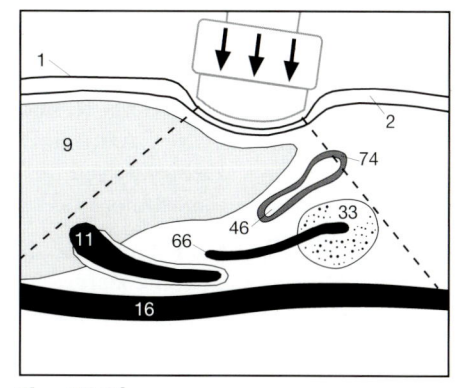

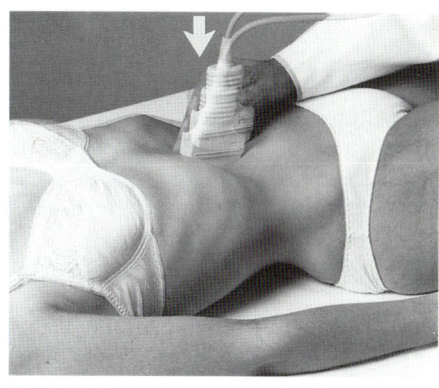

Fig. 79.1 a

Fig. 79.1 b

Fig. 79.2

Competent breathing instructions

Initially, there is some reluctance to tell the patient how to breathe during the examination, though the quality of the sonographic examination of the abdomen strongly depends on the depth of the inspiratory effort necessary, for example, to displace the liver caudally adequate for its visualization. In a neutral respiratory position **(Fig. 79.3 a)**, not only are the liver and spleen obscured by the overlying lung bases, but also the pancreas by an air-containing stomach (26). The low position of the liver (9) in maximum inspiration **(Fig. 79.3 b)** displaces air-containing intestinal loops and stomach (26) inferiorly and opens the pancreatic region (33) for sonographic viewing. The same principle can be applied to facilitate the evaluation of the kidneys. Respiratory maneuvers rarely play a role in the lower abdomen.

Should this approach fail, the stomach can be filled with degassed water (tea), following administration of Buscopan (to eliminate any peristaltic activity). This results in good sound transmission through the stomach. The water should be taken through a straw to avoid inadvertent swallowing of air.

Finally, the examiner can sustain the patient's cooperation better by not only giving instructions to inhale, such as "take a deep breath through your mouth and hold your breath," but also by telling the patient to exhale before overdoing the holding of his or her breath (or after the desired image has been captured by freezing the display). This advice is not as trivial as it seems because the inexperienced examiner often fails to achieve good respiratory cooperation, thereby discouraging the patient and further straining the patient's respiratory condition.

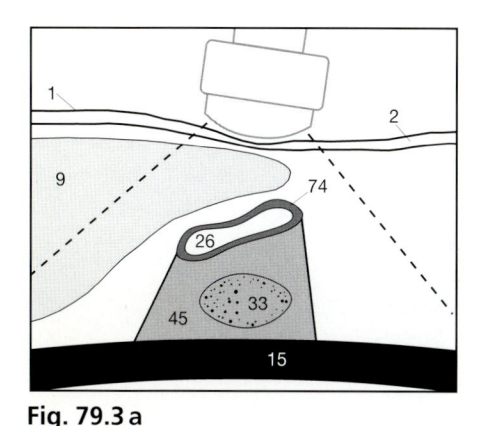

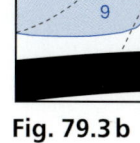

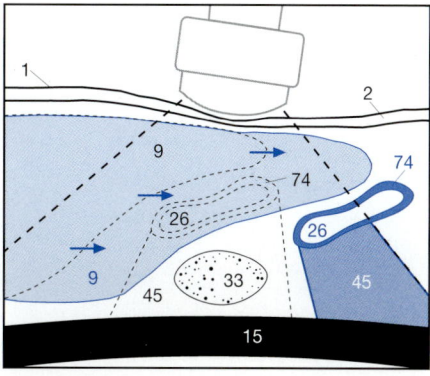

Fig. 79.3 a

Fig. 79.3 b

Acknowledgment

This workbook is intended for physicians, technicians, and medical students who are new to sonography and wish to familiarize themselves with the technique of sonographic image formation and the interpretation of sonographic images. It also takes into consideration the fact that many novices generally have a limited budget for purchasing textbooks on their chosen field.

I therefore thank everybody who contributed to the workbook and strived for a low production cost. The members of Georg Thieme Verlag accommodated all our special requests and wishes concerning the layout of the material, and accompanied and supported the progress of the workbook at all times. Owing to the exceptional engagement and support of Dr. Lüthje, Dr. Bergman, and Mr. Lehnert, the third German edition and the English translation, with Dr. Winter as translator, could be completed in a very short period of time. The Department of Science and Research of North Rhine-Westphalia and Toshiba contributed to the printing costs, making the affordable price a reality.

This interactive workbook is based on the experience I have gathered since 1992 in Düsseldorf as head of the pilot project on medical didactics "Anatomy of Imaging Modalities." The pilot project is gratefully supported by the program "Quality in Teaching" conducted by the Department of Science and Research of North Rhine-Westphalia. The concept of teaching sonography combined with practical exercises in small groups could not have been achieved without the feedback and constructive criticism of the students and pyhsicians in our program and without the continuous cooperation of numerous instructors taken from the ranks of our students. I wish to thank Jörg Kambergs, Andreas Saleh, Ghazaleh Tabatabai, and Jochen Türk, who supported my work for many years and offered valuable suggestions. Furthermore, I wish to mention the willing support of the models Simone Katzwinkel, Wolfgang Bongers, Joana and Würmchen Hofer for the photographs illustrating the positioning of the probe.

I am obliged to Prof. U. Mödder, Prof. H.-G. Hartwig, and Dr. Tanja Reihs for their counsel and for providing several cases. A special note of gratitude goes to my wife Stefanie, who advised me during the planning stage, helped train our assistants, and reviewed the manuscript.

I thank the graphic artists Mrs. Susanne Kniest, and Mrs. Sabine Zarges for their valuable help in drawing all sketches and diagrams, and Mr. Markus Pietrek for the professional photographic displays that demonstrate the handling of the transducer.

Düsseldorf, fall 1998　　　　　　　　　　　　　　Matthias Hofer